KU-005-554

Recent Advances in

Obstetrics and Gynaecology 22

Edited by

John Bonnar MA MD (Hons) FRCOG FRCPI

Emeritus Professor of Obstetrics and Gynaecology, Trinity College,
University of Dublin; Fellow of Trinity College, Dublin;
Trinity Centre for Health Sciences, St James' Hospital, Dublin, Ireland

William Dunlop PhD FRCSEd FRCOG

Professor of Obstetrics and Gynaecology,
School of Surgical and Reproductive Sciences,
University of Newcastle upon Tyne,
Royal Victoria Hospital,
Newcastle upon Tyne, England

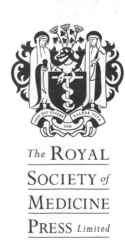

The ROYAL
SOCIETY *of*
MEDICINE
PRESS *Limited*

© 2003 Royal Society of Medicine Press Ltd

1 Wimpole Street, London W1G 0AE, UK

Customers in North America should order via:
RSM Press, c/o Jamco Distribution Inc., 1401 Lakeway Drive, Lewisville, TX 75057, USA. Tel: +1 800 538 1287 (toll free); Fax: +1 972 353 1303. Email: jamco@majors.com

http://www.rsmpress.co.uk/agents.htm

Apart from any fair dealing for the purposes of research or private study, criticism or review, as permitted under the UK Copyright Designs and Patents Act, 1988, no part of this publication may be reproduced, stored or transmitted, in any form or by any means, without the prior permission in writing of the publishers or in the case of reprographic reproduction in accordance of the terms of licences issued by the Copyright Licensing Agency in the UK, or in accordance with the terms of licences issued by the appropriate Reproduction Rights Organization outside the UK. Enquiries concerning reproduction outside the terms stated here should be sent to the publishers at the UK address printed at the top of this page.

The authors are responsible for the scientific content and for the views expressed, which are not necessarily those of the Royal Society of Medicine, or of the Royal Society of Medicine Press Ltd. Medical knowledge is constantly changing. As new information becomes available, changes in treatment, procedures, equipment and the use of drugs become necessary. The editors and the publishers have, as far as possible, taken care to ensure that the information given in this text is accurate and up to date. However, readers are strongly advised to confirm that the information, especially with regard to drug usage, complies with current legislation and standards of practice.

British Library Cataloguing in Publication Data
A catalogue record for this book is available from the British Library

ISBN 1–85315–529–2
ISSN 0143-6848

Commissioning editor - Peter Richardson
Editorial assistant - Gabrielle Lowis
Production by GM & BA Haddock, Midlothian, UK
Printed in Great Britain by Bell & Bain, Glasgow, UK

Recent Advances in

Obstetrics and Gynaecology

22

LIBRARY	
EDUCATION & RESEARCH CENTRE	
WYTHENSHAWE HOSPITAL	
ACC No.	CLASS No.
13625	WQ 100 REC √

Recent Advances in Obstetrics and Gynaecology 21
Edited by John Bonnar

ISBN 0-443-06428 8

ISSN 0143 6848

Contents

Contributors

Katherine J. Barber MB ChB MRCOG
Wellcome Research Fellow, Department of Reproductive and Child Health, University of Birmingham, Birmingham, UK

José L. Bartha MD
Consultant Senior Lecturer, Fetal Medicine Research Unit, University of Bristol, Department of Obstetrics and Gynaecology, St Michael's Hospital, Bristol, UK

Desmond P.J. Barton MD FRCSEd MRCOG FACOG
Consultant Gynaecological Oncologist, The Royal Marsden Hospital, London, UK

Rick D. Clayton MD MRCOG
Fellow in Gynaecological Oncology, The Royal Marsden Hospital, London, UK

Lindsay Cochrane MB ChB MRCOG
Specialist Registrar, Liverpool Women's Hospital, Liverpool, UK

Demetrious L. Economides FRCOG MD
Consultant Obstetrician and Gynaecologist, The Royal Free Hospital School of Medicine, London, UK

John R. Higgins MD FRCPI MRCOG FRANZCOG
Professor, Department of Obstetrics and Gynaecology, University College Cork, Cork, Ireland

Patrick Hogston BSc (Hons) FRCS FRCOG
Consultant Gynaecologist, St Mary's Hospital, Portsmouth, UK

Stuart Jack MRCOG
Specialist Registrar, Department of Gynaecology, Aberdeen Royal Infirmary, Aberdeen, UK

Shehnaaz Jivraj MRCOG
Clinical Research Fellow, Department of Obstetrics and Gynaecology, Faculty of Medicine, Imperial College London, London, UK

Rezan A. Kadir MRCOG FRCS MD
Consultant Obstetrician and Gynaecologist, The Royal Free Hospital School of Medicine, London, UK

Mark D. Kilby MD MRCOG
Professor of Maternal and Fetal Medicine, Department of Fetal Medicine,
Division of Reproduction and Child Health, University of Birmingham,
Birmingham, UK

David E. Parkin MD FRCOG
Consultant Gynaecologist, Department of Gynaecology, Aberdeen Royal
Infirmary, Aberdeen, UK

Bruce McLucas MD
Assistant Clinical Professor, Department of Obstetrics and Gynaecology,
University of California, Los Angeles, School of Medicine, Los Angeles,
California, USA

Deirdre J. Murphy MB BCh BAO DipEpidem MD MRCOG
Professor of Obstetrics and Gynaecology, Honorary Consultant in Obstetrics,
University of Dundee, Dundee, UK

Rajendra S. Rai BSc MD MRCOG
Senior Lecturer/Consultant Gynaecologist, Department of Reproductive
Science and Medicine, Faculty of Medicine, Imperial College of Science,
Technology and Medicine, London, UK

Fiona Reid MB ChB MRCOG
Clinical Research Fellow, The Warrell Unit, St Mary's Hospital, Manchester,
UK

John Reidy FRCR FRCP
Consultant Vascular and Interventional Radiologist, Guy's and St Thomas'
Hospital, London, UK

Michael S. Robson MBBS MRCOG FRCS
Consultant Obstetrician and Gynaecologist, Wycombe General Hospital,
High Wycombe, Buckinghamshire, UK

Joanne Said MB BS MRANZCOG
Clinical Research Fellow in Perinatal Medicine, Department of Perinatal
Medicine, The Royal Women's Hospital and Department of Obstetrics and
Gynaecology, University of Melbourne, Melbourne, Australia

Hassan N. Sallam MB ChB DGO DrChO&G(Alex) FRCOG PhD
Professor in Obstetrics and Gynaecology, The University of Alexandria in
Egypt, and Clinical Director, Alexandria Fertility Center, Alexandria, Egypt

Anthony R.B. Smith MB ChB FRCOG MD
Consultant Gynaecologist, The Warrell Unit, St Mary's Hospital, Manchester,
UK

Peter W. Soothill PhD
Professor of Maternal and Fetal Medicine, University of Bristol, Department
of Clinical Medicine, St Michael's Hospital, Bristol, UK

Stephen A. Walkinshaw BSc MD MRCOG
Consultant in Maternal and Fetal Medicine, Liverpool Women's Hospital,
Liverpool, UK

Shehnaaz Jivraj Rajendra S. Rai

1

Advances in the management of the antiphospholipid syndrome

Antiphospholipid antibodies (aPL) are a heterogeneous family of autoantibodies directed against phospholipid binding plasma proteins. Of this family of approximately 20 antibodies, the two most clinically significant are the lupus anticoagulant (LA) and the anticardiolipin antibodies (aCL). The antiphospholipid syndrome (APS), as originally defined, refers to the association of persistently positive titres of LA or aCL with either arterial and venous thrombosis or recurrent miscarriage or thrombocytopaenia.[1] In the two decades since this description of APS, there has been an explosion of interest in the relationship between aPL and adverse pregnancy outcome at all gestational ages. The current obstetric criteria for the definition of the APS are shown in Table 1.

This review will focus on the laboratory diagnosis of aPL; recent *in vitro* and *in vivo* findings that challenge the currently accepted concepts of aPL-related pregnancy loss and the clinical implications of these findings. We will also discuss the contentious association between aPL and infertility.

LABORATORY DETECTION OF ANTIPHOSPHOLIPID ANTIBODIES

Screening for aPL is subject to widespread inter-laboratory variation. The performance of aPL assays is one of the most controversial issues in laboratory haemostasis. There are several reasons for this. First, the detection of aPL is significantly influenced by 'pre-analytical variables'; second, a variety of assays and instruments are used to detect the same aPL; and finally, longitudinal studies report that the titres of aPL fluctuate over time.

Samples for detection of LA must be taken uncuffed and the sample double-centrifuged within 1 h of venepuncture in order to prepare platelet-poor plasma

Shehnaaz Jivraj MRCOG, Clinical Research Fellow, Department of Obstetrics and Gynaecology, Faculty of Medicine, Imperial College of Science, Technology and Medicine, London, UK

Rajendra S. Rai BSc MD MRCOG, Senior Lecturer/Consultant Gynaecologist, Department of Reproductive Science and Medicine, Faculty of Medicine, St Mary's Campus, Imperial College of Science, Technology and Medicine, Mint Wing, South Wharf Road, London W2 1NY, UK

Table 1 Clinical obstetric criteria for the diagnosis of antiphospholipid syndrome

1. One or more unexplained deaths of a morphologically normal fetus at or beyond the 10th week of gestation, with normal fetal morphology documented by ultrasonography or by direct examination of the fetus

or

2. One or more premature births of a morphologically normal neonate at or before the 34th week of gestation because of severe pre-eclampsia or eclampsia, or severe placental insufficiency

or

3. Three or more unexplained consecutive spontaneous abortions before the 10th week of gestation, with maternal anatomical or hormonal abnormalities and paternal and maternal chromosome causes excluded

for assay. Difficulty in taking the sample or a delay in processing the sample can lead to platelet activation and a false negative result.

No single test will detect all LAs and, ideally, a panel of assays should be performed. In the clinical setting, this is often impractical and, if a single test is to be performed, it should be the dilute Russell's viper venom time (dRVVT), which in a miscarriage population detects LA significantly more often than either the activated partial thromboplastin time (aPTT) or the kaolin clotting time (KCT).[2] It is also imperative to test for both LA and aCL as there is little cross over between positivity for one aPL and another (Fig. 1).

All test results should be confirmed on a repeat sample taken at least 6 weeks later. Individuals may have transiently positive tests which are not thought to be of clinical significance and those with an initial negative test result may be in the transient negative phase of their aPL cycle (Fig. 2).

Advances in the laboratory detection of aPL include the establishment of national reference sera for lupus anticoagulant testing and the development of monoclonal aCL which has rendered aCL testing more uniform.

Antiphospholipid antibodies bind to negatively charged phospholipids, a phenomenon which is dependent on certain co-factors. Prothrombin is a co-factor

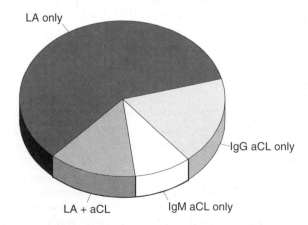

Fig. 1 Distribution of antiphospholipid antibody subtypes in a miscarriage population (*n* = 500).

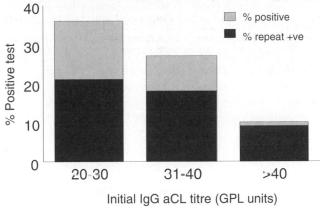

Fig. 2 Testing for anticardiolipin antibodies – transient positivity.

for LA and β_2-glycoprotein I (β_2-GPI), a naturally occurring anticoagulant, is a cofactor for aCL. More recently, evidence is accumulating to suggest a role for anti-β_2-GPI in recurrent miscarriage. A significant proportion of antibodies detected in the conventional aPL assay may be directed against phospholipid-binding proteins such as β_2-GPI rather than against phospholipid itself. The binding of aPL to β_2-GPI inhibits its anticoagulant activity and is thus believed to predispose to thrombosis. A recent case-control study demonstrated that women who experienced unexplained recurrent miscarriage had a significantly higher prevalence of IgA anti-β_2-GPI and IgA aCL antibodies than fertile control women.[3]

MECHANISMS OF PREGNANCY LOSS ASSOCIATED WITH ANTIPHOSPHOLIPID ANTIBODIES

The mechanism of miscarriage and of later pregnancy complications amongst women with the APS has traditionally been ascribed to placental thrombosis which is supported by a considerable body of data. However, thrombosis is not a universal finding and alternative mechanisms of pregnancy loss have been sought. *In vitro* models of implantation have demonstrated that aPL directly impair the function of both the uterine decidua and trophoblast, which may cause an adverse pregnancy outcome.

THROMBOSIS

De Wolf *et al.* reported the first detailed histological examination of a placenta obtained from a woman with an intra-uterine death in association with LA.[4] Macroscopic examination revealed wide-spread areas of placental infarction and microscopic examination showed obliteration of the intervillous blood space. Spiral arteries of the basal plate demonstrated lesions of fibrinoid necrosis, acute atherosis and intraluminal thrombosis. It was inferred that reduced uteroplacental blood flow, as a result of these lesions, led to placental infarction and subsequent fetal death. This initial report was subsequently supported by several individual case and cohort studies.[5]

The mechanism(s) of placental thrombosis associated with aPL remain unclear. However, an attractive mechanism is what has come to be termed the 'annexin hypothesis'. Annexins are soluble, hydrophilic proteins that bind to negatively charged phospholipids in a reversible, calcium-dependent manner. Annexin V is produced by villous trophoblast and, by binding with phospholipids, acts as an anticoagulant in the intervillous space. *In vitro* experiments demonstrate that aPL reduce the levels of annexin V on placental villi thus exposing the intervillous space to thrombosis.[6]

NON-THROMBOTIC PATHOGENESIS OF ANTIPHOSPHOLIPID ANTIBODIES

Placental thrombosis is neither a universal nor a specific finding in aPL pregnancy loss. Recent *in vitro* data, supported by histological evidence, suggest that aPL pregnancy loss is, in some cases, due to defective embryonic implantation and subsequent placentation. Embryonic implantation is a complex process which involves a dialogue between the embryo and the maternal decidua.

Circulating oestrogen and progesterone levels induce morphological changes in the endometrium during the menstrual cycle. Secretory activity in glandular cells and decidualisation of endometrial stromal cells occur in response to activation of progesterone receptors in the luteal phase of the menstrual cycle. When activated, these receptors have the ability to bind consensus DNA and promote transcription. Prolactin (PRL) and insulin growth factor binding protein-1 (IGFBP-1) are examples of genes whose expression increases during progesterone-induced decidualisation in vivo. Mak *et al.* investigated the response of endometrial stromal cells to the monoclonal anticardiolipin antibody ID2.[7] PRL and IGFBP-1 levels were measured after endometrial stromal cells were subjected to a decidualisation stimulus and then exposed to ID2 or an irrelevant antibody. The levels of both PRL and IGFBP-1 were found to be significantly decreased after exposure to ID2 compared with exposure to the control antibody, thereby demonstrating a direct effect of ID2 on endometrial function.

Trophoblast function is also affected by aPL inhibiting syncytialisation, increasing placental apoptosis and impairing trophoblast invasion. Normal placentation requires both extravascular interstitial and endovascular trophoblast invasion of the decidua and maternal spiral arterioles. Replacement of endothelial cells by endovascular trophoblast is preceded by extravascular interstitial modification of the vessel wall by trophoblast. Sebire *et al.* examined products of conception from first trimester miscarriages of 31 aPL positive and 50 aPL negative women with a history of recurrent miscarriage and 20 control women with no history of recurrent miscarriage undergoing surgical termination of pregnancy for non-medical reasons.[8] In no case was significant intervillous or intravascular thrombosis identified. In addition, there was no apparent difference in interstitial extravillous trophoblast invasion. However, **endovascular** trophoblast invasion was seen significantly **less** frequently in aPL-positive cases compared with both aPL-negative cases or controls suggesting that in APS the defect lies more with endovascular trophoblast invasion than intraplacental thrombosis. The mechanism by which aPL affect this process of normal trophoblast invasion may be 3-fold:

1. aPL bind to components on the cell surface of invading trophoblasts and inhibit the function of other cell surface molecules or cause trophoblast damage by activating complement.

2. aPL bind to endothelium of maternal vessels and prevent appropriate trophoblast-endothelium interaction or lead to direct endothelial damage.

3. aPL bind to endovascular trophoblast directly, leading to abnormal formation of endovascular trophoblast plugs.

Recent research in murine models has emphasised fetal regulation of complement activation to modulate potentially damaging maternal immune responses. Complement receptor 1-related gene/protein y (Crry) is a regulatory protein whose role is to block C3 and C4 activation. In the murine model, deficiency of this protein *in utero* is associated with embryonic loss due to the inability of these embryos to suppress spontaneous complement activation and tissue damage mediated by C3. Complement activation may be required for the induction of fetal loss *in vivo* by aPL and, therefore, activation of complement is a critical proximal effector mechanism in aPL-induced fetal injury. In one study, female mice were injected intraperitoneally with either IgG aCL or normal human IgG or saline and, in each group, some mice were injected intraperitoneally with Crry. On day 15 of pregnancy, mice were killed, uteri dissected, fetuses weighed and the presence of fetal resorption sites noted.[9] Treatment with IgG aCL was associated with a significant increase in frequency of fetal resorption and a significant reduction in fetal weight compared with mice treated with IgG aCL and Crry or normal human IgG with or without Crry. In murine models, additional treatment with Crry in the presence of IgG anticardiolipin antibodies appears to cause a reduction in fetal resorption rate and an increase in fetal weight.

The expression of trophoblast adhesions molecules – $\alpha 1$ and $\alpha 5$ integrins, E cadherin and VE cadherin – are also potential targets of aPL action. During placental invasion, the expression of integrin $\alpha 5$ (an inhibitor of invasion) is up-regulated first and then the expression of integrin $\alpha 1$ (a promoter of invasion) is up-regulated next. Cadherins E and VE are two subtypes of the cadherin superfamily, which are differentially expressed during the terminal differentiation of human cytotrophoblasts. These two cadherin subtypes may play discrete roles in the aggregation, differentiation and fusion of villous trophoblast. Di Simone *et al.* investigated the effects, *in vitro*, of aPL on the expression of $\alpha 1$ and $\alpha 5$ integrins and E and VE cadherins by cytotrophoblast cell cultures.[10] Treatment with IgG obtained from a patient with APS significantly decreased $\alpha 1$ integrin and increased $\alpha 5$ integrin expression. IgG aPL down-regulated VE cadherin expression and up-regulated E cadherin expression compared with control IgG or untreated cell cultures. These results suggest that dysfunction of trophoblast invasion, induced by aPL, can be attributed to abnormal expression of trophoblast adhesion molecules.

In addition to impairing trophoblast invasion, aPL impair hormone production by the trophoblast. Di Simone *et al.* reported that hCG secretion was inhibited *in vitro* when gonadotrophin releasing hormone (GnRH) was added to trophoblast cells incubated with aPL containing serum, whereas hCG secretion was increased when GnRH was added to human trophoblast pre-incubated with aPL negative serum.[11] This suggests that aPL could interfere with GnRH-induced signal transduction.

These are all possible, non-thrombotic, mechanisms of aPL pregnancy loss.

RECURRENT MISCARRIAGE AND OBSTETRIC OUTCOME OF ANTIPHOSPHOLIPID SYNDROME

APS is an established cause of recurrent miscarriage. The prevalence of aPL amongst women with recurrent miscarriage (the spontaneous loss of three or more consecutive pregnancies) is 15%.[2] In contrast, the prevalence of these antibodies in a low-risk obstetric population is 2%.[12] The prospective pregnancy outcome of women with APS is poor, with a 90% chance of a further miscarriage in any untreated pregnancy.[13] The majority of miscarriages (94%) occur in the first trimester after the establishment of fetal heart activity.[13]

TREATMENT

A variety of treatment regimens have been used in attempts to improve the poor live-birth rate amongst women with APS (Fig. 3).[14] Low-dose aspirin in combination with heparin remains the only treatment combination that has been demonstrated in two randomised controlled trials to lead to a significant improvement in the live-birth rate.[15,16] This combination remains the first-line treatment of pregnant women with APS.

In a prospective observational study of 150 pregnant APS women treated with aspirin and heparin until 34 completed weeks of gestation, pregnancy-induced hypertension complicated 17% of pregnancies and 24% were delivered before 37 weeks of gestation.[17] In this study, 69% of preterm births occurred at 34–36 weeks. Consequently, there appears to be a relationship between cessation of treatment at 34 completed weeks of gestation and an increase in preterm delivery rate at 34–36 weeks. A randomised trial is currently being undertaken in our unit to determine whether continuing

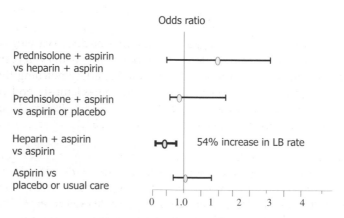

Fig. 3 Meta-analysis of treatment for antiphospholipid syndrome (after Empson *et al.*[14]).

Table 2 Pregnancy outcome according to antiphospholipid subtype

	All women (n = 164)	LA +ve (n = 31)	LA/aCL (n = 12)	IgG aCL (n = 45)	IgM aCL (n = 76)
Proteinuric hypertension	16 (10%)	4 (13%)	2 (17%)	7 (13%)	3 (4%)
Non-proteinuric hypertension	11 (7%)	2 (6%)	1 (8%)	2 (4%)	6 (8%)
Small-for-gestational-age infant	17 (10%)	5 (16%)	4 (33%)	4 (9%)	4 (5%)
Placental abruption	4 (2.4%)	1 (3%)	0	3 (7%)	0
Preterm delivery (< 37 weeks)	21 (13%)	6 (19%)	2 (17%)	8 (18%)	5 (7%)

LA, lupus anticoagulant; aCL, anticardiolipin antibody.

aspirin and heparin treatment until delivery decreases the incidence of late pregnancy complications.

A subsequent study examined the role of uterine artery Doppler to screen for uteroplacental insufficiency amongst pregnant women with APS. The presence of early diastolic notches was assessed and pulsatility indices (PI) measured amongst 170 women with APS (32 with LA only, 47 with IgG aCL, 78 with IgM aCL and 13 with LA and aCL) treated with low-dose aspirin and heparin.[18] Doppler scans were performed twice – at 16–18 weeks and at 22–24 weeks of gestation. The outcome measures assessed were the delivery of a small-for-gestational-age (SGA) infant and the development of pre-eclampsia. Pregnancies associated with LA and IgG aCL had the highest prevalence of complications and those associated with IgM aCL in isolation had the lowest rate of complications (Table 2). Bilateral uterine artery notches were present in 21% and 10% of women at 16 weeks and 24 weeks, respectively, and 26% and 12% of women had unilateral uterine artery notches at 16 weeks and 24 weeks, respectively. A greater proportion of women with LA than with aCL had uterine artery notches and a high PI. In assessing the performance of uterine artery notches and PI as screening modalities for pre-eclampsia and SGA, the same study demonstrated no significant association between uterine artery PI at 16 or 24 weeks and uterine artery notching at 16 weeks in predicting pre-eclampsia or SGA. Amongst women with LA, bilateral uterine artery notches at 24 weeks predicted pre-eclampsia (likelihood ratio 12.8 for positive test and 0.27 for negative test result) and SGA infants (likelihood ratio 13.6 for positive test and 0.2 for negative test result.) Uterine artery notching at 22–24 weeks did not predict pre-eclampsia or SGA in pregnancies associated with IgG aCL or IgM aCL. The authors suggest that this may be due to varying severity of the disease process affected by different subtypes of aPL, with LA representing the most severe end of the spectrum. Bilateral uterine artery notching therefore appears to be a promising screening modality for pre-eclampsia and SGA in women with LA. However, future larger studies (45 women in this study had LA) are needed to confirm this finding before Doppler screening can be recommended as routine for women with LA.

More recently, questions have been raised about the role of both aspirin and heparin in improving pregnancy outcome in women with APS. One small, double-blind, randomised controlled trial of 75 mg aspirin *versus* placebo in women with aPL, failed to demonstrate a difference in live-birth rate.[19] The other study, purporting to be a randomised, controlled study of aspirin *versus* aspirin and heparin amongst women with APS, reported no additional benefit to be gained by the use of heparin.[20] Both studies can be criticised for their design, laboratory assays, randomisation and interpretation.

In the study by Farquharson *et al.*, the high live-birth rates, the low incidence of perinatal complications and lack of benefit of heparin reported are entirely expected as the majority of participants in this study did not satisfy the laboratory criteria to be diagnosed as having APS.[20] The study design also limits the value of the data. Randomisation took place at up to 12 weeks' gestation, yet data from the authors' own unit show that after 8 weeks' gestation the live-birth rate in on-going pregnancies is 98%.[21] Clearly, a number of women destined to have a successful pregnancy were included. Twenty-four women (a quarter of the study cohort) switched treatment arm, but no details as to the gestational age at which the switch occurred is provided.

In our recurrent miscarriage clinic, women with a diagnosis of the APS are commenced on 75 mg aspirin once daily as soon the urine pregnancy test is positive. When an intra-uterine pregnancy is confirmed on transvaginal ultrasound scan, low molecular weight heparin is commenced. A platelet count is checked every 2–4 weeks to screen for thrombocytopaenia, a rare side-effect of heparin administration. Women are followed up fortnightly during the first trimester in an early pregnancy clinic where ultrasound scans are done and where they are seen by clinic staff to maintain continuity of care. Both aspirin and heparin are continued until 34 completed weeks of gestation.

WOMEN REFRACTORY TO ASPIRIN AND HEPARIN

Although the combined use of aspirin and heparin results in a high live-birth rate, there is a cohort of women refractory to this treatment combination. Consequently, alternative therapeutic modalities are currently under investigation. One such modality is intravenous immunoglobulin (IVIG); the rationale for use is the anti-idiotypic down-regulation of auto-antibody production. The only randomised controlled study of the use of IVIG amongst pregnant women with aPL was of insufficient power to determine any difference in live-birth rates between IVIG and combination treatment with aspirin and heparin ($n = 16$).[22] The preterm delivery rate and birth weight were similar in the two groups, but fewer cases of intra-uterine growth restriction (IUGR) and neonatal intensive care unit (NICU) admissions were seen in the group given IVIG although the differences were not statistically significant (IUGR:IVIG, 0% *versus* placebo 33%; NICU:IVIG, 20% *versus* placebo 44%). This suggested a possible beneficial effect of IVIG. However, until well-designed, randomised, controlled trials of sufficient power are conducted, IVIG is best reserved for cases refractory to treatment with aspirin and heparin.

OSTEOPAENIA AND LONG-TERM HEPARIN THERAPY

Osteopaenia is a major concern of long-term heparin therapy. Heparin appears to act as a chelating agent with binding to calcium ions resulting in secondary hyperparathyroidism. This enhances bone resorption by directly impeding osteoblast activity and enhancing osteoclast activity with effects on the skeleton by disturbing the bone matrix mucopolysaccharides leading to defective ossification.[23,24] Results of several clinical studies have shown that long-term treatment with heparin during pregnancy results in a reduction of bone mineral density (BMD). However, studies have also shown that a reduction in bone mineral density occurs in untreated pregnancies as well.[25,26]

In a prospective study of 123 women treated with aspirin and heparin for APS, dual photon X-ray absorptiometry (DEXA) was used to measure BMD at the lumbar spine (L2–L4), the neck of femur and the forearm at 12 weeks of gestation (baseline), immediately post partum (within 2 weeks of delivery) and 12 weeks' post partum.[27] In this study, 46 women took unfractionated heparin and 77 women took low molecular weight heparin. Overall, there was a significant decrease in the BMD at both the lumbar spine (3.7%; $P < 0.001$) and at the neck of femur (0.9%; $P = 0.007$), but not at the forearm between 12 weeks of gestation and immediately post partum. No significant difference in BMD changes during pregnancy was found between those women receiving unfractionated heparin and those receiving low molecular weight heparin. The results of this large study were similar to those of prospective studies of BMD changes in untreated pregnancies.[25,26] The same study also found that 8% of women were osteopaenic at the lumbar spine at 12 weeks' gestation indicating that a considerable proportion of women have low bone density prior to pregnancy. In addition, women who breast fed were found to have significantly lower BMD compared to women who did not breast feed.

Women requiring thromboprophylaxis during pregnancy can, therefore, be re-assured that loss in BMD of the lumbar spine associated with the use of heparin as thromboprophylaxis during pregnancy is similar to that which occurs physiologically during untreated pregnancies.

ANTIPHOSPHOLIPID ANTIBODIES AND INFERTILITY

The role of aPL in failure of successful implantation after IVF by embryo transfer (IVF-ET) is a matter of controversy. Some authors report that circulating aPL may be responsible for implantation failure whereas others cast doubt on this opinion. A recent review of published data demonstrated that most studies have reported an increased prevalence of aPL among women undergoing IVF-ET.[28] However, prospective studies examining the effect of aPL on the outcome of IVF-ET demon-strate that aPL do not significantly affect implantation and on-going pregnancy rates.[29] The increased prevalence of aPL among women with infertility may, therefore, be part of a generalised autoimmune disturbance associated with infertility.

A prospective observational study of 380 women attending our unit who were undergoing their first IVF cycle, reported that although the prevalence of aPL (aCL or LA) was higher in the population referred for IVF-ET compared with a normal fertile population (23% *versus* 2%; $P < 0.05$), there was no significant difference in the future viable pregnancy rate (9% *versus* 12.4%; $P = 0.45$) or live-birth rate (9% *versus* 12%; $P = 0.57$) in women who were aPL positive and aPL negative, respectively.[30]

Routine screening for aPL among women undergoing IVF-ET is not warranted and therapeutic interventions should be used only in well-designed, randomised, controlled trials.

CONCLUSIONS

Recent *in vitro* data challenges the concept of aPL pregnancy loss being purely thrombotic in origin. Emphasis is now placed on the deleterious effects of these antibodies on embryonic implantation.

Aspirin in combination with heparin remains the treatment of choice for pregnant women with APS. Successful pregnancies are characterised by a high incidence of pre-eclampsia, intra-uterine growth restriction and preterm labour. Future research should be aimed at assessing the optimum duration and timing of the dose of heparin.

Further experience with aspirin and heparin therapy has shown a cohort of women with APS who are resistant to this treatment. Intravenous immunoglobulin is a promising therapy but, until randomised controlled studies of sufficient power to determine efficacy are conducted, this treatment should only be used in the context of a clinical trial.

Key points for clinical practice

- Laboratory testing for aPL (aCL and LA) should be done according to internationally agreed standardised guidelines.

- Although thrombosis is frequently observed in the decidual and placental vasculature of women with APS, this finding is neither universal nor specific to aPL pregnancies.

- Recent evidence suggests that aPL impair both decidua and trophoblast function via mechanisms unrelated to thrombosis.

- The established treatment for pregnant women with APS is aspirin (75 mg daily) as soon as a urinary pregnancy test is positive and either unfractionated subcutaneous heparin (5000 IU, 12-hourly) or low molecular weight heparin (Enoxaparin 20 mg once daily) until 34 completed weeks of pregnancy.

- Treated pregnancies amongst women with APS remain at-risk for pregnancy-induced hypertension, intra-uterine growth restriction and preterm labour. These pregnancies should be managed in a unit with specialist obstetric and neonatal intensive care facilities.

- Use of heparin in prophylactic doses during pregnancy is not associated with significant loss of bone mineral density over and above that which occurs physiologically in untreated pregnancies.

- Routine screening for aPL in women undergoing IVF-ET is not warranted.

- Intravenous immunoglobulin at present is best reserved for cases refractory to treatment with aspirin/heparin in the context of a controlled clinical trial.

References

1. Hughes GR. Thrombosis, abortion, cerebral disease, and the lupus anticoagulant. *BMJ* 1983; **287**: 1088–1089.

2. Rai RS, Regan L, Clifford K *et al*. Antiphospholipid antibodies and beta2-glycoprotein-I in 500 women with recurrent miscarriage: results of a comprehensive screening approach. *Hum Reprod* 1995; **10**: 2001–2005.
3. Lee RM, Branch DW, Silver RM. Immunoglobulin A anti-beta2-glycoprotein antibodies in women who experience unexplained recurrent spontaneous abortion and unexplained fetal death. *Am J Obstet Gynecol* 2001; **185**: 748–753.
4. De Wolf F, Carreras LO, Moerman P, Vermylen J, Van Assche A, Renaer M. Decidual vasculopathy and extensive placental infarction in a patient with repeated thromboembolic accidents, recurrent fetal loss, and a lupus anticoagulant. *Am J Obstet Gynecol* 1982; **142**: 829–834.
5. Sebire NJ, Backos M, Goldin RD, Regan L. Placental massive perivillous fibrin deposition associated with antiphospholipid antibody syndrome. *Br J Obstet Gynaecol* 2002; **109**: 570–573.
6. Rand JH, Wu XX, Andree HA *et al*. Pregnancy loss in the antiphospholipid-antibody syndrome – a possible thrombogenic mechanism. *N Engl J Med* 1997; **337**: 154–160.
7. Mak IY, Brosens JJ, Christian M *et al*. Regulated expression of signal transducer and activator of transcription, Stat5, and its enhancement of PRL expression in human endometrial stromal cells *in vitro*. *J Clin Endocrinol Metab* 2002; **87**: 2581–2588.
8. Sebire NJ, Fox H, Backos M, Rai R, Paterson C, Regan L. Defective endovascular trophoblast invasion in primary antiphospholipid antibody syndrome-associated early pregnancy failure. *Hum Reprod* 2002; **17**: 1067–1071.
9. Holers VM, Girardi G, Mo L *et al*. Complement C3 activation is required for antiphospholipid antibody-induced fetal loss. *J Exp Med* 2002; **195**: 211–220.
10. Di Simone N, Castellani R, Caliandro D, Caruso A. Antiphospholipid antibodies regulate the expression of trophoblast cell adhesion molecules. *Fertil Steril* 2002; **77**: 805–811.
11. Di Simone N, De Carolis S, Lanzone A, Ronsisvalle E, Giannice R, Caruso A. *In vitro* effect of antiphospholipid antibody-containing sera on basal and gonadotrophin releasing hormone-dependent human chorionic gonadotrophin release by cultured trophoblast cells. *Placenta* 1995; **16**: 75–83.
12. Lockwood CJ, Romero R, Clyne LP, Coster B, Hobbins JC. The prevalence and biologic significance of lupus anticoagulant and anticardiolipin antibodies in general obstetric population. *Am J Obstet Gynecol* 1989; **161**: 369–373.
13. Rai RS, Clifford K, Cohen H, Regan L. High prospective fetal loss rate in untreated pregnancies of women with recurrent miscarriage and antiphospholipid antibodies. *Hum Reprod* 1995; **10**: 3301–3304.
14. Empson M, Lassere M, Craig JC, Scott JR. Recurrent pregnancy loss with antiphospholipid antibody: a systematic review of therapeutic trials. *Obstet Gynecol* 2002; **99**: 135–144.
15. Kutteh WH. Antiphospholipid antibody-associated recurrent pregnancy loss: treatment with heparin and low-dose aspirin is superior to low-dose aspirin alone. *Am J Obstet Gynecol* 1996; **174**: 1584–1589.
16. Rai R, Cohen H, Dave M, Regan L. Randomised controlled trial of aspirin and aspirin plus heparin in pregnant women with recurrent miscarriage associated with phospholipid antibodies (or antiphospholipid antibodies). *BMJ* 1997; **314**: 253–257.
17. Backos M, Rai R, Baxter N, Chilcott IT, Cohen H, Regan L. Pregnancy complications in women with recurrent miscarriage associated with antiphospholipid antibodies treated with low dose aspirin and heparin. *Br J Obstet Gynaecol* 1999; **106**: 102–107.
18. Venkat-Raman N, Backos M, Teoh TG, Lo WT, Regan L. Uterine artery Doppler in predicting pregnancy outcome in women with antiphospholipid syndrome. *Obstet Gynecol* 2001; **98**: 235–242.
19. Pattison NS, Chamley LW, Birdsall M, Zanderigo AM, Liddell HS, McDougall J. Does aspirin have a role in improving pregnancy outcome for women with the antiphospholipid syndrome? A randomized controlled trial. *Am J Obstet Gynecol* 2000; **183**: 1008–1012.
20. Farquharson R, Quenby S, Greaves M. Antiphospholipid syndrome in pregnancy: a randomized, controlled trial of treatment. *Obstet Gynecol* 2002; **100**: 408–413.
21. Brigham SA, Conlon C, Farquharson RG. A longitudinal study of pregnancy outcome following idiopathic recurrent miscarriage. *Hum Reprod* 1999; **14**: 2868–2871.

22. Branch DW, Peaceman AM, Druzin M *et al*. A multicenter, placebo-controlled pilot study of intravenous immune globulin treatment of antiphospholipid syndrome during pregnancy. The Pregnancy Loss Study Group. *Am J Obstet Gynecol* 2000; **182**: 122–127.
23. Dahlman TC, Sjoberg HE, Ringertz H. Bone mineral density during long-term prophylaxis with heparin in pregnancy. *Am J Obstet Gynecol* 1994; **170**: 1315–1320.
24. De Swiet M, Dorrington Ward P, Fidler J *et al*. Prolonged heparin therapy in pregnancy causes bone demineralisation. *Br J Obstet Gynaecol* 1983; **90**: 1129–1134.
25. Khastgir G, Studd JWW, King H *et al*. Changes in bone density and biochemical markers of bone turnover in pregnancy-associated osteoporosis. *Br J Obstet Gynaecol* 1996; **103**: 716–718.
26. Shefras J, Farquharson RG. Bone density studies in pregnant women receiving heparin. *Eur J Obstet Gynecol Reprod Biol* 1996; **65**: 171–174.
27. Backos M, Rai R, Thomas E, Murphy M, Dore C, Regan L. Bone density changes in pregnant women treated with heparin: a prospective, longitudinal study. *Hum Reprod* 1999; **14**: 2876–2880.
28. Backos M, Rai R, Regan L. Antiphospholipid antibodies and infertility. *Hum Fertil* 2002; **5**: 35–36.
29. Hornstein MD, Davis OK, Massey JB, Paulson RJ, Collins JA. Antiphospholipid antibodies and *in vitro* fertilization success: a meta-analysis. *Fertil Steril* 2000; **73**: 330–333.
30. Chilcott IT, Margara R, Cohen H *et al*. Pregnancy outcome is not affected by antiphospholipid antibody status in women referred for *in vitro* fertilization. *Fertil Steril* 2000; **73**: 526–530.

John R. Higgins Joanne Said

2

The clinical implications of thrombophilia in pregnancy

The term thrombophilia has been used to describe a number of conditions that predispose to vascular thrombosis.[1] The term encompasses both inherited and acquired disorders of haemostasis. The focus of this chapter is the emerging role of the inherited thrombophilias in human pregnancy. This group of disorders came to prominence in the non-pregnant population with the observation that a significant proportion of patients with venous thromboembolism carry inherited defects in their haemostatic system. The association between pregnancy-related venous thromboembolism and inherited thrombophilias has now also been confirmed.[2,3] Perhaps of more significance is the recent recognition of possible associations between the inherited thrombophilias and several important pregnancy complications including pre-eclampsia, fetal growth restriction (FGR), placental abruption and stillbirth. The putative common pathophysiology suggested to link these disorders with the inherited thrombophilias is excessive uteroplacental vascular thrombosis. Measuring the strength of these associations and unravelling the underlying pathophysiological mechanisms are now key research challenges for all those involved in the care of pregnant women.[4]

NORMAL PREGNANCY

The coagulation system, normally in equilibrium with a delicate balance between procoagulant clotting factors, naturally occurring anticoagulants and fibrinolytic factors, is shifted in pregnancy in favour of the procoagulant side.[5] This adaptation may have evolutionary advantages in terms of protecting the mother from postpartum haemorrhage, a significant cause of obstetric mortality;

John R. Higgins MD FRCPI MRCOG FRANZCOG, Professor, Department of Obstetrics and Gynaecology, University College Cork, Ernville Hospital, Cork, Ireland (for correspondence)

Joanne Said MB BS MRANZCOG, Clinical Research Fellow in Perinatal Medicine, Department of Perinatal Medicine, The Royal Women's Hospital and Department of Obstetrics and Gynaecology, University of Melbourne, Melbourne, Australia however, it also places the woman in danger of developing life-threatening vascular thrombosis during the antenatal and postpartum period.[6] Pregnant women are at a 5–6-fold increased risk of developing venous thrombo-embolism during pregnancy simply due to the fact that they are pregnant.[6]

Various physiological changes in the coagulation system in the systemic circulation have been described during pregnancy.[5] Important among these are: (i) increase in naturally occurring clotting factors (including Factor VIII, von Willebrand's Factor, Factor V, fibrinogen); (ii) decrease in naturally occurring anticoagulants. (particularly protein S); (iii) acquired resistance to activated protein C; and (iv) impaired fibrinolytic activity due to increases in the expression of the plasminogen activator inhibitor 1 and 2 genes (PAI 2 comes in large part from the placenta[5]).

The limited data available from the uteroplacental circulation suggest that, in this circulation, the coagulation system is even further activated with a reactive increase in fibrinolysis.[7] This makes the uteroplacental circulation particularly vulnerable to an additional insult such as the presence of an inherited thrombophilia which may lead to excessive thrombosis.

INHERITED THROMBOPHILIA

The inherited thrombophilias that are currently tested for clinically are a heterogeneous group of conditions which vary in their prevalence, thrombogenic potential, and clinical significance. In clinical terms, they can be divided into two broad groups as shown in Table 1. As a 'rule-of-thumb', the prevalence of the disorder is inversely proportional to the thrombogenic potential. The prevalence of thrombophilia in different ethnic groups varies widely. A high prevalence of the Factor V Leiden mutation has been identified in Northern European countries while the prothrombin gene mutation is more common in patients with a Southern European background.[1] The currently identified thrombophilias appear to be far less common in patients of African and Asian backgrounds.

Recently, mutations in the thrombomodulin gene[8,9] the plasminogen activator inhibitor gene,[10] and a further mutation in the Factor V gene (the Factor V Cambridge mutation)[11] have been investigated. There is no doubt that, with the rapid development in laboratory methodologies, further thrombophilias will be identified.[12] In addition, the development of real-time PCR technology and the automation of DNA extraction and preparation

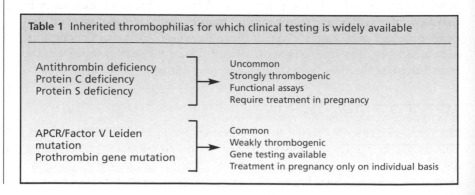

Table 1 Inherited thrombophilias for which clinical testing is widely available

Antithrombin deficiency Protein C deficiency Protein S deficiency	Uncommon Strongly thrombogenic Functional assays Require treatment in pregnancy
APCR/Factor V Leiden mutation Prothrombin gene mutation	Common Weakly thrombogenic Gene testing available Treatment in pregnancy only on individual basis

techniques will mean that testing for these types of genetic defects will become very inexpensive and widely available. The current group of inherited thrombophilias are described in more detail below.

ANTITHROMBIN

Antithrombin is a naturally occurring anticoagulant and acts as the primary inhibitor of thrombin.[1] Antithrombin binds to thrombin thereby preventing the conversion of fibrinogen to fibrin by thrombin.[1] Antithrombin has two important binding sites – a thrombin binding site and a heparin binding site. The binding of heparin to antithrombin increases the anticoagulant activity of antithrombin by approximately 1000-fold.[1]

Many mutations have been identified in the gene encoding antithrombin.[13] These mutations can result in either a reduction in the quantity of normal antithrombin or production of normal amounts of abnormal antithrombin. These defects are referred to as type I and type II defects, respectively.[13] The risk of venous thrombosis has been shown to correlate well with the absolute quantity of antithrombin in patients with type I antithrombin deficiency, and the site of the mutation in patients with type II defects; mutations occurring in the thrombin binding site carry a greater risk than mutations at the heparin binding site.[13]

The prevalence of antithrombin deficiency has been estimated at about 0.02%[14] and the condition is generally inherited as an autosomal dominant trait.[15] Patients with antithrombin deficiency have been estimated to have a 50-fold increased life-time risk of venous thromboembolism making antithrombin deficiency one of the most potent thrombophilias.[1] Because of the very large number of mutations possible in the antithrombin gene, functional, clot-based assays are generally used to assess antithrombin deficiency.[13]. Previous small studies have not demonstrated any significant change in antithrombin levels during pregnancy; however, premenopausal women and women using combined oral contraceptives have been shown to have slightly lower levels.[16]

PROTEIN C

Protein C circulates as an inactive precursor and requires activation by thrombin to exert its anticoagulant effects.[1] Protein C also requires the presence of Protein S to act as a co-factor.[1] Once activated, Protein C binds to and inactivates Factors Va and VIIIa (Fig. 1). The prevalence of Protein C deficiency in the general population is approximately 0.3%.[17] As Protein C deficiency is also associated with multiple genetic polymorphisms,[15] laboratory testing also relies on clot-based assays. Type I (quantitative reduction of functionally normal protein) and type II (production of abnormal protein) defects have been described.[15]

ACTIVATED PROTEIN C RESISTANCE/FACTOR V LEIDEN MUTATION

The Factor V Leiden mutation is a single point mutation at nucleotide 1691. This mutation results in the substitution of the amino acid glutamine for arginine at amino acid 506 in the Factor V protein,[18] thereby abolishing the cleavage site for activated Protein C making Factor V resistant to the action of

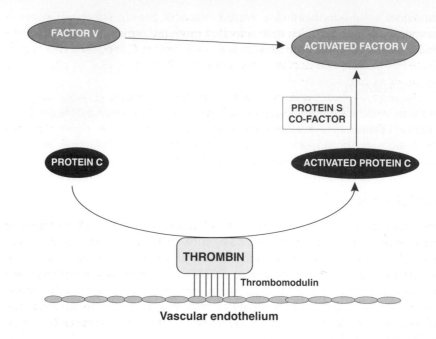

Fig. 1 Activation of Protein C by thrombin. Activated Protein C then binds to and inhibits activated Factor V.

activated Protein C. The general population prevalence of the Factor V Leiden mutation varies significantly with ethnicity, being more common in people of Northern European extraction (prevalence up to 10–15%)[15] than those of Japanese or Afro-American extraction (prevalence about 1–3%). Heterozygosity for the Factor V Leiden mutation has been associated with a 3–8-fold increase in the risk of venous thromboembolism in pregnancy.[18]

In non-pregnant populations, 90–95% of cases of activated Protein C resistance are associated with the Factor V Leiden mutation. Up to a further 5% can be attributed to a more recently described mutation – the Factor V Cambridge mutation.[11] This is a mutation occurring at the 306 APC cleavage site. Co-inheritance of both the Factor V Leiden and Factor V Cambridge mutations may predispose to an increased risk of venous thromboembolism above that of Factor V Leiden alone.

Acquired activated Protein C resistance is also seen during pregnancy. Resistance to activated Protein C increases as pregnancy progresses.[20] Pregnancies complicated by pre-eclampsia are also associated with increased resistance to activated Protein C. The mechanism for this change is uncertain, but is possibly secondary to the reduction in Protein S levels as well as the increase in Factor V levels seen in pregnancy. Several studies have reported that Protein C levels do not change in pregnancy.[20]

PROTEIN S

Protein S is also a vitamin K dependent protein that functions as a co-factor for activated Protein C in binding to and inactivating Factor Va.[15] The precise mechanism of action in this regard remains uncertain, but may be a membrane-bound complex with activated Protein C which renders Factors Va and VIIIa more easily accessible to activated Protein C mediated cleavage.[15]. Some 60% of Protein S circulates bound to the C4b binding protein whereas the remainder circulates free.[15]

The large number of different genetic polymorphisms mean that the diagnosis of Protein S deficiency is dependent on functional, clot-based assays. Estimates of Protein S deficiency in the population have been difficult to establish. Protein S levels are significantly reduced in pregnancy.[1] The risks of VTE with inherited Protein S deficiency has been estimated to increase between 2–10-fold.[1]

PROTHROMBIN GENE

Prothrombin is the inactive precursor of thrombin.[1] A G-to-A mutation at nucleotide 20210 in the prothrombin gene has been described, that results in excessive production of prothrombin and hence increased circulating prothrombin levels.[19] Like the Factor V Leiden mutation, this mutation shows significant ethnic variation, being most prevalent in Southern European populations with an overall population prevalence of 2–3%. The increased risk of venous thromboembolism in association with this mutation has been estimated at 2–3-fold.[1]

HYPERHOMOCYSTEINAEMIA

Homocysteine is an intermediate by-product formed during the metabolism of methionine. It is metabolised to form cysteine via the transulphuration pathway or can be converted back to methionine via the re-methylation pathway.[21] Homocysteine is thought to exert a toxic effect on the haemostatic system perhaps indirectly by its effects on the endothelium through generation of hydrogen peroxides, depletion of nitric oxide mediated detoxification of homocysteine, and impairing endothelial cell thrombomodulin expression.[22]

Modest elevations of homocysteine have been described in association with inherited polymorphisms of the methylenetetrahydrofolate reductase (MTHFR) gene, as well as the environmental deficiencies of folate and vitamin B_{12}. The C-to-T mutation at nucleotide 677 in the gene encoding the MTHFR enzyme has been described[21] which, in the homozygous form, results in the production of a thermolabile variant of the MTHFR enzyme. This has a functional activity of only about 30% and results in modest elevations of homocysteine that can be reversed with relative ease by an increase in dietary folic acid. Up to 15% of a Caucasian population are heterozygous for this mutation.[22] The increased risk of venous thromboembolism has been estimated at about 2–3-fold.[15]

Another mutation in the MTHFR gene has been identified more recently. The A-to-C mutation at nucleotide 1298 occurs in the presumed regulatory domain of this gene.[23] Whether this mutation is associated directly with an increased risk of venous thromboembolism is uncertain; however, it may well be associated with a more severe phenotypic expression in patients who also carry the 677 polymorphism.[23] As the gene encoding the MTHFR enzyme is quite large, further polymorphisms may be identified which will help to explain the differences seen in the phenotypic expression.

CLINICAL FEATURES OF THROMBOPHILIAS IN PREGNANCY

VENOUS THROMBOEMBOLISM

The incidence of venous thromboembolism (VTE) in pregnancy has been estimated in several large studies. McColl et al.[24] reported on 72,201 deliveries over an 11-year period at two Glasgow hospitals. Only objectively confirmed thromboses were included and an incidence of 0.86 per 1000 deliveries was identified. Lindqvist et al.[25] reported an incidence of 1.3 per 1000 in patients studied in Sweden over a 3-year period. The increase in the rate found in the study by Lindqvist and colleagues may be attributable to an improved level of ascertainment possible in Sweden through centralisation of hospital records. Both studies confirmed an even distribution of antepartum and postpartum events and, in antepartum events, a fairly even distribution across each trimester.

The contribution of thrombophilia to pregnancy-related thromboembolism has been studied by Gerhardt et al.[2] In a case-control study of 119 women with venous thromboembolism and 233 age-matched controls, the prevalence of the Factor V Leiden mutation in women with venous thromboembolism was 43.7% compared to only 7.7% in women without a history of venous thromboembolism, giving a relative risk of developing venous thromboembolism in carriers of the Factor V Leiden mutation of 9.3 (95% CI, 5.1–16.9). Likewise, the relative risk of developing venous thromboembolism in carriers of the prothrombin mutation was calculated at 15.2 (95% CI, 4.2–52.6). Of particular importance was the finding that 9.3% of the patients with venous thromboembolism carried both the Factor V Leiden and the prothrombin gene mutation. None of the women without thrombotic events were carriers of both mutations. Based on the prevalence of Factor V Leiden and prothrombin gene mutations in the general population, the expected prevalence of such a combination was calculated at 0.10%. This gave an estimated relative risk of 107 for developing venous thromboembolism in patients who carry the combination of mutations. Using a regression model and assuming a background rate of venous thromboembolism in pregnancy of 1 in 1500, they calculated that a carrier of Factor V Leiden mutation has a 1 in 500 risk of VTE , a carrier of the prothrombin gene mutation has a risk of 1 in 200 and a carrier of both mutations has a risk of VTE in pregnancy of approximately 1 in 20.

By contrast, the MTHFR mutation was not found to be strongly associated with venous thromboembolism, occurring in 9.6% of women with a history of venous thromboembolism compared to 9.4% of women without such a history; however, the MTHFR genotype was seen more commonly in women with venous thromboembolism in the puerperium than during pregnancy. Possibly, the effects of antenatal folate supplementation may have caused this skewed effect.

Grandone[3] also reported an increased risk of pregnancy-related venous thromboembolism in carriers of thrombophilia, with the relative risk for carriers of Factor V Leiden estimated at 16.3 (95% CI, 4.8–54.9), that of prothrombin 10.2 (95% CI, 4.0–25.9) and that of the MTHFR mutation 2.1 (95% CI, 1.0–4.5). These figures clearly provide useful information for the clinician when counselling patients with thrombophilia about the increased risks of venous thromboembolism during pregnancy.

THROMBOPHILIA AND PREGNANCY COMPLICATIONS

Pregnancy complications such as severe pre-eclampsia, fetal growth restriction, placental abruption and unexplained stillbirth continue to represent major causes of perinatal and maternal morbidity and mortality. The precise aetiology of these conditions remains uncertain; however, the frequent association between these conditions and the histopathological finding of placental infarction and thrombosis in the uteroplacental circulation[26-30]suggests that factors leading to excessive thrombosis in the uteroplacental circulation may play an important aetiological role. With respect to the inherited thrombophilias, the association with pre-eclampsia has been the focus of most interest.

In 1995, Dekker et al.[31] reported on the high prevalence of thrombophilia in patients with severe, early-onset pre-eclampsia. In this uncontrolled study, 24.7% of patients with severe pre-eclampsia had Protein S deficiency, 16% had APCR and 17.7% had hyperhomocysteinaemia. This contrasted with the background population prevalence for these abnormalities (Protein S, 0.2–2%; APCR, 3–7%; hyperhomocysteinaemia, 2–3%). In addition, anticardiolipin antibodies were identified in 29.9% of patients with severe, early-onset pre-eclampsia. (estimated population prevalence 1–3%). Subsequent studies[32-34] have also demonstrated that patients with severe pre-eclampsia have between 2–3 times the risk of carrying an inherited thrombophilia compared to those without pre-eclampsia. In a case-control study performed in Israel, Kupferminc et al.[32] reported that 35 of 63 women (56%) with severe pre-eclampsia had one of the following thrombophilic mutations: Factor V Leiden (heterozygous or homozygous), prothrombin gene mutation (hetero-zygous or homozygous) or MTHFR 677 homozygous. By contrast, only 24 of 126 control women (19%) had the same thrombophilic mutations. Of particular interest was the finding that 7 women with severe pre-eclampsia had combined thrombophilias whereas none of the women without pre-eclampsia had more than one thrombophilia.

In the only prospective study to date, Lindqvist[18] was unable to demonstrate a significant association between the Factor V Leiden mutation and pregnancy complications. Of women with pregnancy complications, 11.1% were identified with the mutation compared to only 9.8% of those without pregnancy complications. This higher prevalence of the Factor V Leiden mutation is characteristic of the Northern European country in which this study took place. The possible advantage of the Factor V Leiden mutation in reducing postpartum haemorrhage was, however, confirmed with a reduction of intrapartum and postpartum haemorrhage to 3.7% in those who were heterozygous or homozygous for the Factor V Leiden mutation compared to 7.9% in those who did not carry the mutation. We have not found significant associations between pre-eclampsia (in both pre-eclamptic pedigrees and sporadic cases) and several different inherited thrombophilic markers.[35-37] The current information suggests that the associations between the inherited thrombophilias and pre-eclampsia are strongest with severe, early-onset pre-eclampsia and still poorly defined with the more common clinical presentations of pre-eclampsia.

FGR, FETAL LOSS AND PLACENTAL ABRUPTION

The frequent pathological findings of infarction, and uteroplacental thrombosis in placentae from pregnancies complicated by FGR,[26] suggest again a possible mechanism for the relationship between the inherited thrombophilias and FGR. In a case-control study performed in Israel,[32] FGR was seen twice as frequently in patients with severe pre-eclampsia and thrombophilia compared to those with pre-eclampsia without thrombophilia. This suggests that women with pre-eclampsia and thrombophilia may express a more severe form of the pre-eclampsia spectrum, with possibly a greater degree of placental thrombosis.

The association between placental abruption and thrombophilia has been demonstrated in several studies.[38,39] Kupferminc et al.[38] found a highly significant association between placental abruption and the prothrombin gene mutation. In a systematic review, Alfirevic et al.[40] found that there was a significant relationship between placental abruption and the Factor V Leiden mutation, OR 6.7 (95% CI, 2.0–21.6) for heterozygous carriers and OR16.9 (95% CI, 2.0–141.9) for homozygous carriers, the prothrombin mutation OR 28.9 (95% CI, 3.5–236.7), hyperhomocysteinaemia OR 3.5 (95% CI, 1.5–8.1) and activated Protein C resistance OR 6.6 (95% CI, 2.3–19.0).

In an early study on the association between fetal loss and inherited thrombophilia, Preston et al.[41] reported on the findings from the European Prospective Cohort on Thrombophilia (EPCOT). This large cohort involved 843 women with thrombophilia, of whom 571 had 1524 pregnancies. A control group was made up of genetically unrelated partners or acquaintances of the index cases. The risk of fetal loss (of any type) amongst women with thrombophilia was found to be 1.35 times greater than in women without thrombophilia (95% CI, 1.01–1.82). When stillbirth and miscarriage were examined separately, the odds ratio was much higher for stillbirth at 3.6 (95% CI, 1.4–9.4) compared to 1.27 (95% CI, 0.94–1.71) for miscarriage. When the relationship between individual thrombophilias and fetal loss was examined, the strongest association was again seen where there was a combination of defects. No statistically significant association was seen between Factor V Leiden and miscarriage or stillbirth; however, several subsequent studies[42,43] have reported an increased risk of fetal loss in association with Factor V Leiden. The contribution of thrombophilia to miscarriage remains controversial.[44] What is borne out in numerous studies, however, is that combinations of defects appear to increase the risk and hence, testing for all the known thrombophilias may yield more information than testing for one alone.

The data currently available do not allow accurate assessment of the association between the individual pregnancy complications and the individual thrombophilias. McLintock et al.[45] in a recent review used pooled data from all published or presented research. While not as meaningful as a

Table 2 Low molecular weight heparin (LMWH) dosage schedule

LMWH	Therapeutic dose	Prophylactic dose
Dalteparin (Fragmin)	100 U/kg twice daily	5000 U daily
Enoxaparin (Clexane)	1 mg/kg twice daily or 1.5 mg/kg daily	40 mg daily
Tinzaparin (Innohep)	175 IU/kg daily	4500 IU daily or 75 IU/kg

large prospective study, some estimate of the strength of the associations becomes possible. For instance, the pooled odds ratio for placental abruption and MTHFR C667T was 2.7 (95% CI, 1.4–5.0), for Factor V Leiden was 4.6 (95% CI, 2.0–10.3), and for prothrombin gene mutation was 7.6 (95% CI, 2.8–21).

TREATMENT

The advent of low molecular weight heparin (LMWH) has transformed the issue of long-term anticoagulation in pregnancy. Previously, unfractionated heparin administered subcutaneously was the mainstay of treatment. LMWHs have several important advantages over unfractionated heparin including a more predictable therapeutic response, increased bioavailability, longer half-life, reduced incidence of heparin-induced thrombocytopenia and of heparin-induced osteoporosis and much less need for laboratory monitoring. These advantages are of particular benefit in pregnancy. Thus, when considering the risks and benefits of anticoagulation treatment in an individual pregnant patient, the potential complications of treatment have diminished significantly.

A proposed dosage schedule is shown in Table 2. The intensity of monitoring is still being defined. Regular assessment of platelet count with perhaps a baseline measurement pre-treatment and further measurements a week after commencing treatment and monthly thereafter is important to exclude the development of thrombocytopenia. The activated partial thromboplastin time (APTT) used to monitor unfractionated heparin is less influenced by the administration of LMWH. Anti-Xa levels are the most useful measure of pharmacological effect of the LMWHs; however, in the non-pregnant population, because of the consistency of response with LMWHs, they are generally not utilised.[46] With alterations in renal clearance of heparins likely to occur as pregnancy progresses, there are rational reasons to use anti-Xa levels at least until more wide-spread clinical experience is available. Recent guidelines from the British Society for Haematology[46] suggest measuring the peak anti-Xa activity after the first month of use and then 4–6 weekly to ensure that the therapeutic window is achieved and not exceeded. These guidelines recommend aiming for a peak plasma anti Xa level of 0.35–0.5 when measured by a chromogenic substrate assay 3 h postinjection. In contrast, the 2001 Australasian guidelines[47] advised no necessity for anti-Xa monitoring. With the increasing use of LMWH, obstetricians need to become informed and competent with prescribing LMWH.

Women being treated during pregnancy should be aware of the need to manage labour and delivery carefully. In particular, they should know of the increased risks of spinal haematoma with regional anaesthesia. Women taking prophylactic doses of LMWH should be instructed to omit their daily dose if they have any symptoms of labour. An interval of more than 20 h from the last dose should allow the insertion of a regional block without significant increased risk.[47] An epidural catheter can be removed 12–20 h after placement and the next injection delayed until 4 h after removal.[47] Prophylactic doses can be recommenced within 6 h of delivery. To ensure the choice of epidural anaesthesia is available, induction of labour can be offered with the dose of LMWH being omitted on the morning of induction. In women being treated in the first month after an acute venous thrombo-embolic event, the options are to switch to intravenous unfractionated heparin for 24–36 h before induction

Table 3 Recommendations for anticoagulant prophylaxis to prevent venous thromboembolism in women with thrombophilias during pregnancy

Thrombosis history	Antithrombin deficiency	Protein C deficiency	Protein S deficiency	FVL or PGM homozygous	FVL or PGM heterozygous
Personal history of VTE independent of family history	ThA	PrA	PrA	PrA	Negot
Family history of VTE in one or more first degree relatives	ThA/PrA	PrA	PrA	PrA	Negot
Family history of VTE in a distant relative	ThA/PrA	PrA	Negot	Negot	Nil
No personal or family history of VTE	ThA/PrA	PrA	Nil	Nil	Nil

FVL, Factor V Leiden mutation; PGM, prothrombin gene mutation; ThA, therapeutic anti-coagulation recommended throughout pregnancy and puerperium due to the very high risk of venous thromboembolism; PrA, prophylactic anticoagulation recommended throughout pregnancy and puerperium; Negot, need for prophylaxis negotiable on a case-by-case basis until further data become available; Nil, postpartum prophylaxis or no prophylaxis.

and cease treatment at the onset of labour or to change to prophylactic LMWH for 24–36 h before intervention. The aim should be to ensure that no woman delivers while being therapeutically anticoagulated. In the absence of any other indication, vaginal birth is the preferred mode of delivery.

In women with inherited thrombophilia, who should be offered treatment? Despite the importance of VTE in pregnancy as a major cause of maternal morbidity and mortality, the low incidence of VTE requires large intervention trials. Consensus guidelines and protocols[46,47] form the basis of treatment. This approach is based on risk assessment for each patient depending on the thrombogenic potential of an individual thrombophilia, the patient's personal and family history of VTE and other specific risk factors such as obesity, smoking and surgical delivery. Recently published Australian guidelines provide a basis for management (Table 3).[47]

Much of the work on the role of anticoagulation in preventing pregnancy complications in patients with thrombophilia is extrapolated from the existing research demonstrating improvements in perinatal outcome for patients with antiphospholipid syndrome and recurrent miscarriage who are treated antenatally with heparin and aspirin.[48] Whether we can safely base our assumptions on these data is uncertain since the antiphospholipid syndrome is thought to exert its effects, in part, through uteroplacental thrombosis, but also through as yet undefined immune-mediated pathways.

Several small studies comparing pregnancies treated with heparin to those without have suggested a small improvement in perinatal outcome;[49,50] however, most of the improvement appears to be seen in the first trimester with no major improvements seen in obstetric complications beyond this time. Transient improvements in Doppler blood flows in the uterine arteries have been demonstrated following heparin use;[51] however, this did not equate to any improvements in clinical outcome. Uncertainty remains, therefore, in what constitutes appropriate treatment for patients who are otherwise asymptomatic but found through testing of family members to carry an inherited thrombophilia. The answer to this question no doubt lies in the results of further prospective studies examining the relationship of pregnancy complications and thrombophilia in patients who have no other potential risk factors as well as large, multicentred, randomised, controlled trials comparing the various antithrombotic treatments.

Aspirin still remains a possible treatment modality. A recent systematic review[52] reported that antiplatelet agents are associated with a 15% reduction in the rate of pre-eclampsia in women at risk. Possibly, women with thrombophilia constitute such an at-risk group. Again the potential role of aspirin in women with inherited thrombophilias remains to be determined.

Folic acid supplementation can lead to correction of raised homocysteine levels in women with mild hyperhomocysteinaemia.[22] In the absence of clinical outcome data, it seems reasonable that women with hyperhomocysteinaemia becoming pregnant should be treated with folic acid supplements throughout pregnancy.

TESTING FOR THROMBOPHILIA

Screening for the inherited thrombophilias after an obstetric complication has already become wide-spread despite the uncertainties about the strength of the associations and the benefits of anti-thrombotic therapy in future pregnancies. Ideally, women should only be screened in the context of rigorous controlled intervention trials. In the absence of such trials, it would be prudent if three basic criteria are met before screening for inherited thrombophilias after an obstetric complication: (i) patients are counselled as to the current clinical uncertainty in this area and are aware of the implications for family members of a positive screen; (ii) a referral pathway to a haematologist for the patient and her family is available; and (iii) the clinician ordering the test has, in consultation with the patient, a treatment/management plan in place for future pregnancies.

The place of screening in patients with venous thromboembolism is well established and is part of the work-up in a patient who suffers a spontaneous event in pregnancy.[46] Studies have indicated that up to 50% of these patients will be shown to carry one of the identified thrombophilias.[2,3] Testing can be safely deferred until after anticoagulation is completed since the presence or absence of a thrombophilic marker is unlikely to alter the duration or intensity of treatment for the acute event.[46] Testing the patient remote from the clinical event is also more likely to yield a more accurate result since the acute event is often associated with alterations in antithrombin and Protein C function. When testing is undertaken, the tests in Table 4 should be included.

Screening patients for thrombophilia following pregnancy complications is now commonly performed by many obstetricians based on the accumulating evidence of an association between complications and thrombophilia.[38-40] The biggest challenge with this approach is in deciding precisely what to do with these results – both the positive and the negative results. In many situations, the interventions for patients with pregnancy complications but without thrombophilic markers will be much the same as those with thrombophilic markers.

Table 4 Testing for inherited thrombophilia

Antithrombin

Chromogenic assay – levels unchanged in pregnancy, decreased in pre-eclampsia

Protein C

Levels unchanged in pregnancy, affected by warfarin therapy

Free and total Protein S

Levels much decreased in pregnancy, affected by warfarin therapy

Activated Protein C resistance/Factor V Leiden

Testing for the Factor V Leiden mutation should be undertaken if activated Protein C resistance is detected. DNA testing can also be used during pregnancy where APCR is common in the latter half of pregnancy

Prothrombin gene mutation

There is no functional test for this mutation

Fasting homocysteine levels

If elevated, check vitamin B_{12} levels and methionine loading test. Further testing may include the MTHFR C667T mutation

Currently, no evidence supports screening asymptomatic patients at the commencement of pregnancy or prior to oral contraceptive use. Screening in this situation is expensive and time consuming and carries a very low yield.[5]

The importance of re-testing patients who are known to have a thrombophilia or who have had episodes of venous thromboembolism or pregnancy complications without a thrombophilic marker should be emphasised. There is now very good evidence that combinations of thrombophilias carry a cumulative risk for both venous thromboembolism as well as pregnancy complications. Because new thrombophilias are being described, we must ensure that patients are tested for the up-to-date panel of thrombophilias.

CONCLUSIONS

The associations between thrombophilia and important obstetric complications is not proof of 'cause-and-effect'. However, the common uteroplacental pathology of excessive thrombosis in these complications provides biological plausibility and the apparent 'dose-response relationship' in that carriage of two thrombophilic markers, or homozygosity for a mutation is associated with a higher risk of obstetric complications, suggest an aetiological role. Clearly, many women with inherited thrombophilia do not develop pregnancy complications. Likewise, not all women with pregnancy complications carry a thrombophilic marker. Large observational studies, basic laboratory research and multicentred, controlled trials of antithrombotic therapy are required to improve the counselling and treatment of pregnant women with inherited thrombophilia.

References

1. Walker ID, Thrombophilia in pregnancy. *J Clin Pathol* 2000; **53**: 573–580.

Key points for clinical practice

- The inherited thrombophilias are a heterogeneous group of disorders which need to be considered as distinct clinical entities.

- The prevalence of an inherited thrombophilia is roughly inversely proportional to its thrombogenic potential.

- Important ethnic differences are found in prevalence.

- Gene testing for inherited thrombophilias is becoming easier and cheaper.

- Screening for the inherited thrombophilias is now an established part of the investigation and management of venous thromboembolism in non-pregnant and pregnant populations.

- Low molecular weight heparins appear to be significantly easier to use, reliable and safer than unfractionated heparin in pregnancy. Many pregnant women are likely to receive such therapies and obstetricians need to be informed and competent in prescribing them.

- The role of the inherited thrombophilias in the aetiology and pathogenesis of many important pregnancy complications is uncertain. The strength of these associations and the benefits of anti-thrombotic therapy in future pregnancy are still unclear.

- Despite the uncertainty testing for inherited thrombophilias appears to be widespread after obstetric complications. If testing is being performed, three basic criteria should be met: (i) patients are counselled as to the current clinical uncertainty in this area and are aware of the implications for family members of a positive screen; (ii) a pre-existing referral pathway to a haematologist for the patient and her family is available; and (iii) the clinician ordering the test has, in consultation with the patient, a treatment/management plan in place for future pregnancies.

2. Gerhardt A, Scharf RE, Beckman MW *et al*. Prothrombin and Factor V mutations in women with a history of thrombosis during the puerperium. *N Engl J Med* 2000; **340**: 374–380.
3. Grandone E, Margaglione M, Colazzo D *et al*. Genetic susceptibility to pregnancy related venous thromboembolism: roles of Factor V Leiden, prothrombin G20210A and methylenetetrahydrofolate reductase C677T mutations. *Am J Obstet Gynecol* 1998; **179**: 1324–1328.
4. Higgins JR. Pregnancy and the impact of inherited thrombophilias. *Aust NZ J Obstet Gynaecol* 2000; **40**: 118–121.
5. Greer IA. Thrombosis in pregnancy. Maternal and fetal issues. *Lancet* 1999; **353**: 1258–1265.
6. ACOG Practice Bulletin. Thromboembolism in pregnancy. *Int J Gynaecol Obstet* 2001; 203–212.
7. Higgins JR, Walshe JJ, Darling MR, Norris L, Bonnar J. Haemostasis in the uteroplacental and peripheral circulations in normotensive and pre-eclamptic pregnancies. *Am J Obstet Gynecol* 1998; **179**: 520–526.
8. Nakabayashi M, Yamamoto S, Suzuki K. Analysis of thrombomodulin gene polymorphism in women with severe early onset pre-eclampsia. *Semin Thromb Hemost* 2002; **25**: 473–479.

9. Franchi F, Biguzzi E, Cetin I et al. Mutations in the thrombomodulin and endothelial Protein C receptor genes in women with late fetal loss. Br J Haematol 2001; 114: 641–646.

10. Glueck CJ, Kupferminc MJ, Fontaine RN, Wang P, Weksler BB, Eldor A. Genetic hypofibrinolysis in complicated pregnancies. Obstet Gynecol 2001; 97: 44–48.

11. Williamson D, Brown K, Luddington R, Baglin I. Factor V Cambridge: a new mutation (ARG-306-THR) associated with the resistance to activated Protein C. Blood 1998; 91: 1140–1144.

12. Bertina RM. Genetic approach to thrombophilia Thromb Haemost 2001; 86: 92–103.

13. Lane DA, Olds RJ, Boisclair M et al. Antithrombin III mutation database: first update. Thromb Haemost 1993; 70: 361–369.

14. Tait RC, Walker ID, Perry DJ et al. Prevalence of antithrombin deficiency in the healthy population. Br J Haematol 1994; 87: 106–112.

15. De Stefano V, Finazzi G, Manucci PM. Inherited thrombophilia. Pathogenesis, clinical syndromes and management. Blood 1996; 87: 3531–3544.

16. Tait RC, Walker ID, Islam SIAM et al. Influence of demographic factors on antithrombin activity in a healthy population. Br J Haematol 1993; 84: 476–478.

17. Tait RC, Walker ID, Reitsma PH et al. Prevalence of Protein C deficiency in the healthy population. Thromb Haemost 1995; 73: 87–93.

18. Lindqvist PG, Svenson PJ, Mars K, Grennert L, Luterkort M, Dahlback B. Activated Protein C resistance (FV: Q506) and pregnancy. Thromb Haemost 1999; 81: 532–537.

19. Poort SR, Rosendaal FR, Reitsma PH et al. A common genetic variation in the 3' untranslated region of the prothrombin gene is associated with elevated plasma prothrombin levels and an increase in venous thrombosis. Blood 1996; 88: 3698–3703.

20. Mimuro S, Lahoud R, Beutler L, Trudinger B. Changes of resistance to activated Protein C in the course of pregnancy and prevalence of the Factor V Leiden mutation. Aust NZ J Obstet Gynaecol 1998; 38: 200–204.

21. Frosst P, Blom HJ, Milos R et al. A candidate genetic risk factor for vascular disease: a common mutation in methylenetetrahydrofolate reductase. Nat Genet 1995; 10: 111–113.

22. Welch GN, Loscalzo J. Homocysteine and atherothrombosis. N Engl J Med 1998; 338: 1042–1050.

23. Isotalo PA, Wells GA, Donnelly GA. Neonatal and fetal methylenetetrahydrofolate reductase genetic polymorphisms: an examination of C677T and A1298C mutations. Am J Hum Genet 2000; 67: 986–990.

24. McColl MD, Ramsay JE, Tait RC. Risk factors for pregnancy associated thromboembolism. Thromb Haemost 1997; 78: 1183–1188.

25. Lindqvist P, Dahlbäck B, Marsél K. Thrombotic risk during pregnancy: a population study. Obstet Gynecol 1999; 96: 595–599.

26. Salafia C, Minor VK, Pezzullo JC, Popek EJ, Rosenkrantz TS, Vintzileas AM. Intrauterine growth restriction in infants of less than thirty-two weeks gestation: associated placental pathologic features. Am J Obstet Gynecol 1995; 173: 1049–1057.

27. Ghidini A, Salafia C, Pezzullo JC. Placental vascular lesions and likelihood of diagnosis of pre-eclampsia. Obstet Gynecol 1997; 90: 542–545.

28. Salafia CM, Pezzullo JC, Lopez-Zeno JA, Simmens S, Minuer VK, Vintziteon AM. Placental pathologic features of preterm pre-eclampsia. Am J Obstet Gynecol 1995; 173: 1097–1105.

29. Many A, Schreiber L, Rosner S, Lessing JB, Eldor AE, Kupferminc MJ. Pathologic features of the placenta in women with severe pregnancy complications and thrombophilia. Obstet Gynecol 2001; 98: 1041–1044.

30. Arias F, Romero R, Joist H, Kraus FT. Thrombophilia: a mechanism of disease in women with adverse pregnancy outcome and thrombotic lesions of the placenta. J Matern Fetal Med 1998; 7: 277–286.

31. Dekkar GA, de Vries JIP, Doelitzsch PM et al. Underlying disorders associated with severe early-onset pre-eclampsia. Am J Obstet Gynecol 1995; 173: 1042–1048.

32. Kupferminc MG, Fait G, Many A, Gordon D, Eldor A, Lessing JB. Severe pre-eclampsia and high frequency of genetic thrombophilic mutations. Obstet Gynecol 2000; 96: 145–149.

33. Lindoff C, Ingemarsson I, Martinsson G, Segelmark M, Thysell H, Astedt B. Pre-eclampsia is associated with a reduced response to activated Protein C. Am J Obstet Gynecol 1997; 176: 457–460.

34. von Tempelhof GF, Heilmann L, Spanuth E, Kunzmann E, Hommel G. Incidence of the Factor V Leiden mutation, coagulation inhibitor deficiency and elevated antiphospholipid antibodies in patients with pre-eclampsia or HELLP syndrome. *Thromb Res* 2000; **100**: 363–365.
35. Higgins JR, Kaiser T, Moses EK, North R, Brennecke SP. Prothrombin G20210A mutation. Is it associated with pre-eclampsia? *Gynaecol Obstet Invest* 2000; **50**: 254–257.
36. Kaiser T, Brennecke SP, Moses EK. C677T methylenetetrahydrofolate reductase polymorphism is not a risk factor for pre-eclampsia/eclampsia among Australian women. *Hum Hered* 2001; **51**: 20–22.
37. Borg A, Higgins JR, Brennecke SP, Moses EK. Thrombomodulin Ala 455 Val dimorphism is not associated with pre-eclampsia in Australian and New Zealand women. *Gynaecol Obstet Invest* 2002; In press.
38. Kupferminc MJ, Eldor A, Steinman N *et al*. Increased frequency of genetic thrombophilia in women with complications of pregnancy. *N Engl J Med* 1999; **340**: 9–13.
39. Alfirevic Z, Moussa HA, Martlew V, Briscoe L, Perez-Cascal M, Toh CH. Postnatal screening for thrombophilia in women with severe pregnancy complications. *Obstet Gynecol* 2001; **97**: 753–759.
40. Alfirevic Z, Roberts D, Martlew V. How strong is the association between maternal thrombophilia and adverse pregnancy outcome? A systematic review. *Eur J Obstet Gynaecol Reprod Biol* 2002; **101**: 6–14.
41. Preston FE, Rosendaal FR, Walker ID *et al*. Increased fetal loss in women with heritable thrombophilia. *Lancet* 1996; **348**: 913–916.
42. Brenner B, Sang G, Weiner Z, Younis J, Blumenfield Z, Lanir N. Thrombophilic polymorphisms are common in women with fetal loss without apparent cause. *Thromb Haemost* 1999; **82**: 6–9.
43. Barè SN, Pòka R, Balogh I, Ajzner È. Factor V Leiden as a risk factor for miscarriage and reduced fertility. *Aust NZ J Obstet Gynaecol* 2000; **40**: 186–190.
44. Blumenfield Z, Brenner B. Thrombophilia-associated pregnancy wastage. *Fertil Steril* 1999; **72**: 765–774.
45. McLintock C, North RA, Dekkar G. Inherited thrombophilias: implications for pregnancy-associated venous thromboembolism and obstetric complications. *Curr Probl Obstet Gynaecol Fertil* 2001; **24**: 114–149.
46. Walker ID, Greaves M, Preston FE. Guideline. Investigation and management of heritable thrombophilia. *Br J Haematol* 2001; **114**: 512–528.
47. Hague WM, North RA, Gallus AS *et al*. A Working Group on behalf of the Obstetric Medicine Group of Australasia. Anticoagulation in pregnancy and the puerperium. *Med J Aust* 2001; **175**: 258–263.
48. Rai R, Cohen H, Dave M, Regan L. Randomised controlled trial of aspirin and aspirin plus heparin in pregnant women with recurrent miscarriage associated with phospholipid antibodies (or antiphospholipid antibodies). *BMJ* 1997; **314**: 253–257.
49. Riyazi N, Leeda M, de Vries JIP, Huigjens PC, van Geijn HP, Dekkar GA. Low-molecular-weight heparin combined with aspirin in pregnant women with thrombophilia and a history of pre-eclampsia or fetal growth restriction: a preliminary study. *Eur J Obstet Gynaecol Reprod Biol* 1998; **80**: 49–54.
50. Brenner B, Hoffman R, Blumenfield Z *et al*. Gestational outcome in thrombophilic women with recurrent pregnancy loss treated by enoxaparin. *Thromb Haemost* 2000; **83**: 693–697.
51. Bar J, Mashiah R, Cohen-Sacher B *et al*. Effect of thromboprophylaxis on uterine and fetal circulations in pregnant women with a history of pregnancy complications. *Thromb Res* 2001; **101**: 235–241.
52. Duly L, Henderson-Smart D, Knight M, King J. Antiplatelet drugs for the prevention of pre-eclampsia and its consequences: a systematic review. *BMJ* 2001; **322**: 329–333.

José L. Bartha Peter W. Soothill

3

Clinical applications of fetal therapy

Fetal therapy could be considered as any intervention that may benefit a fetal condition diagnosed prenatally, but that concept is so wide and would include so many existing different procedures as to be unhelpful. For example, prophylactic measures (like anti-D globulin for Rhesus disease or corticosteroids for fetal lung maturation), actions during labour in cases of suspected fetal hypoxia (Caesarean section, amnio-infusion, tocolysis) and medical and surgical treatments on the mother (treatment of perinatal infections, nutrient supplementation) could all be included.

The application of evidence-based medicine to fetal therapy is limited at present. The rarity of many of the conditions in which fetal therapy is used often makes randomised studies impractical, and so meta-analysis or systematic reviews are not possible. Observational studies have demonstrated significant improvements in the outcomes in some clinical situations after prenatal diagnosis and therapy. Fetal therapy is currently entering a new era of larger and more wide-spread implementation and evidence-based evaluation.

This chapter concentrates on those conditions and interventions that seem to have clear clinical benefit and brief mention of the others.

TRANSFUSION THERAPY IN HAEMATOLOGICAL CONDITIONS

FETAL ANAEMIA

Intra-uterine intraperitoneal transfusion, was originally described by Liley,[1] mainly in fetuses with hydrops and low gestational age, and was associated

José L. Bartha MD, Consultant Senior Lecturer, Fetal Medicine Research Unit, University of Bristol, Department of Obstetrics and Gynaecology, St Michael's Hospital, Southwell Street, Bristol BS2 8SR, UK

Peter W. Soothill PhD, Professor of Maternal and Fetal Medicine, University of Bristol, Department of Clinical Medicine, St Michael's Hospital, Southwell Street, Bristol BS2 8EG, UK (for correspondence)

with a poor survival rate. To improve the outcomes, Rodeck et al.[2] designed a new procedure based on intravascular transfusion under the direct vision of fetoscopy. However, this procedure also had a high risk for fetal loss. In the early 1980s, Bang et al.[3] described a new method of umbilical cord needling under ultrasound guidance. The procedure was widely developed during the 1980s and is currently the first choice for intravascular access.

Fetal transfusion is undertaken by puncturing the umbilical vein, usually at placental cord insertion, with a 20–22-gauge needle after local anaesthesia in the maternal abdominal wall. Some centres use paralyzing agents such as vecuronium to stop fetal movements when sampling intrafetal vessels but, in our experience, this is rarely needed. A sample of fetal blood is obtained to determine the pretransfusion haemoglobin concentration. Adult blood, irradiated (to prevent graft versus host rejection) and packed to a hematocrit of 75–85% (to reduce volume), is used. Some authors have used maternal blood as the source of red cells in order to obtain theoretical benefits in terms of decreasing the risk for sensitization to new red-cell antigens,[4] but this has not been demonstrated to be beneficial. The amount of blood to be transfused to restore the haemoglobin concentration back to normal can be calculated by applying established mathematical formulae, often using computer programmes. During transfusion, the visualization of the turbulence caused by the injected blood entering the umbilical vein confirms that the blood is being infused correctly. The volume needed is given as fast as possible without causing a bradycardia since the placenta seems to help the fetus to manage this blood volume expansion.

Transfusions are repeated depending on the rate of hematocrit drop. The use of non-invasive techniques, such as middle cerebral artery Doppler,[4] to predict fetal haemoglobin concentrations facilitates the timing of the next transfusion. Using intra-uterine intravascular transfusions, the overall survival rate is about 84%,[6] reaching near 100% in cases of non-hydropic fetuses. Before the era of intra-uterine transfusion, an immunized woman had a 50% chance of losing her baby, the effect of the clinical application of fetal therapy in this field is clear.[7]

Parvo-virus B19 infection can also cause a severe fetal anaemia leading, in the most severe cases, to fetal hydrops and death. The virus causes arrest of maturation of red blood cell precursors at the late normoblast stage and also a decrease in the number of platelets. In addition, myocarditis leading to heart failure may contribute to the development of fetal hydrops. Reported data suggest a benefit of transfusion therapy over conservative management in infected fetuses especially in severe cases.[8]

FETAL THOMBOCYTOPENIA

In allo-immune thrombocytopenia, fetal platelets are destroyed by maternal antibodies directed against platelet antigens, mainly HPA-1a or HPA-5a. In the affected neonates, 10–20% develop intracranial haemorrhage, with 25–50% of these occurring prenatally.[9] Investigation is often by fetal blood sampling at 18–22 weeks which may be repeated at 28–32 weeks if the fetus is not seriously affected earlier. Therapeutic options include maternal administration of intravascular immunoglobulin, corticosteroid therapy and fetal platelet transfusion. The latter may also be used prophylactically at each fetal blood sampling to avoid bleeding during the procedure. However, the transfused platelet life-span is only about 4–5 days and weekly transfusions may be needed to control the disease. Cumulative risk for fetal loss of serial weekly transfusions is approximately 6% per pregnancy, which indicates the need for development of less invasive approaches.[10]

The relative risk reduction in mortality with antenatal therapy is 57% (95% CI, 0.19–0.77).[11] Treatment of pregnancies with intravenous immunoglobulin increased the likelihood of a neurologically normal outcome, with a relative risk of 1.68 (95% CI, 1.3–2.2), and treatment of pregnancies with only antenatal platelet transfusions increased the likelihood of a neurologically normal outcome with a relative risk of 1.63 (95% CI, 1.1–2.1). Further studies are needed to determine the relative roles of fetal platelet transfusions and maternal administration of immunoglobulin in the perinatal outcomes. Because fetal blood sampling is difficult before 20 weeks, in cases at risk of very early fetal intracranial haemorrhage (*i.e.* where a sibling has suffered an intracranial haemorrhage prior to 20 weeks), treatment of the mother with intravenous immunoglobulin (1 g/kg/week or more) seems justifiable from around 16 weeks' gestation.[12]

TWIN-TO-TWIN TRANSFUSION SYNDROME

Twin-to-twin transfusion syndrome (TTTS) is a condition that affects 5–15% of all pregnancies with monochorionic placentae and is associated with a very high risk of perinatal mortality and morbidity. A number of treatments have been introduced to treat the condition. Several randomised studies are ongoing, but so far no clear evidence is available from randomised trials to influence practice.[13] Classically, the perinatal survival of TTTS pregnancies managed without *in utero* procedures has been low (around 30%) and the mortality rate in groups of very severe cases may reach 100%. Fetal therapy is associated with survival rates of about 70–80% varying according to the procedure, gestational age at diagnosis, severity, *etc.*

AMNIODRAINAGE

Amniodrainage has been used not only for the treatment of TTTS but also for relieving maternal symptoms in women with severe polyhydramnios of other aetiology. Criteria for amniotic fluid reduction are amniotic fluid index greater than 40 cm or the deepest single pool greater than 12 cm, but the decision is often best determined by maternal discomfort or possibly by maternal and fetal condition in cases of TTTS. Amniotic fluid usually re-accumulates quickly, and the procedure needs to be repeated frequently. Each 100 ml of amniotic fluid removed decreases the amniotic fluid index about 1 cm.[14] Using this guide, the amount of fluid to be removed can be calculated.

Serial amnioreduction is one of the most commonly used methods for treating TTTS. Early, aggressive amniocentesis may have the capability to alter interfetal blood flow, possibly as a result of changes in intravascular pressure, which are related to changes in intra-amniotic pressure.[15] The standard procedure consists of passing a 19-gauge needle into the amniotic cavity under local anaesthesia and amniotic fluid is drained with a syringe system until the deepest amniotic fluid pool is less than 8 cm. Another more rapid and radical technique has been reported using vacuum bottle system and aspirating considerable more volume of amniotic fluid with possibly even better outcomes.[16]

LASER THERAPY

Fetoscopic laser placental vessel ablation was originally described by DeLia et al. in 1990.[17] Several series[18,19] have demonstrated that the interruption of vascular anastomoses between monochorionic twins can dramatically improve the outcomes particularly in early-onset cases where the prognosis is otherwise very poor. Survival rates for at least one twin reach 70–80% and, unlike amniodrainage and septostomy, the procedure seems to reduce abnormal neurological sequelae in the survivors. Unsolved questions remain: (i) what to do in cases of anterior placenta; (ii) how to identify vessels feeding not only superficial but also deep anastomoses; and (iii) ways to recognise which anastomoses are truly participating in the process. In most cases of monochorionic twins, these anastomoses may help to compensate the asymmetric placental vascular supply that normally exists.[20] The procedure is not free of complications both from the laser coagulation of vessels which sometimes can produce severe bleeding leading to fetal death, and from the endoscopic procedure which includes preterm labour, premature rupture of membranes, etc.

SEPTOSTOMY

Deliberate puncture of the amniotic membranes to cause a leak, and so equilibration, of the amniotic sac volumes has been suggested to be associated with survival rates better than, or comparable to, more invasive modalities.[21] The prolongation of pregnancy from diagnosis to delivery has been reported as significantly better for those treated by septostomy compared to amnioreduction.[22] The logic behind this approach is hard to understand, but one explanation is that the restoration of amniotic fluid in the donor sac may allow fetal drinking and so rehydration. Certainly, at the appropriate gestational age, fetal lung development might be improved.

CORD LIGATION OR COAGULATION

Several procedures have been described for cord occlusion in cases of acardiac twin. Some of them may also be used in cases of twin-to-twin transfusion syndrome in which one of the fetuses is so severely damaged that death would be expected soon. In these cases, cord occlusion may prevent severe brain injury in the surviving twin as a consequence of the death of its co-twin with the placental anastomoses. A wide variety of procedures has been reported, such as alcohol injection, bipolar coagulation, endoscopic laser, ultrasound-guided interstitial laser,[23] and cord clamping; bipolar diathermy is probably the best.[24]

SHUNTS

FETAL THERAPY FOR OBSTRUCTIVE UROPATHY

The clinical outcomes of renal dysplasia and pulmonary hypoplasia in neonates with posterior urethral valves or with other causes of obstructive uropathy lead to a neonatal mortality of about 45%. Since these complications are related to the duration and the degree of the obstruction, an early and permanent relief of the obstruction can ameliorate the effects.

Vesico-amniotic shunting became wide-spread but, after the analysis of the International Fetal Surgery Registry[25] showing procedure-related mortality of 4.7% and rates of only 41% for overall survival, the method received some severe criticisms. This reaction against the procedure still persists mainly in some paediatric urologists. The issues giving rise to concern were the lack of experienced and technically skilled operators to perform the procedure, the wide spectrum of the underlying causes, the lack of any patient selection criteria and consistent outcome measurements.[26] After that study, the only series that addressed the efficacy of prenatal decompression in the treatment of fetal obstructive uropathy[27] reported a higher survival rate in those who underwent prenatal intervention.

Selection criteria are based mainly on detailed ultrasound examination which includes amniotic fluid volume, assessment of urinary tract, appearance of kidneys (renal cysts, hyperechogenic kidneys) and the existence of other abnormalities. Measurements of urinary electrolytes and β_2-microglobulin are used to select patients with the best prognosis to recover normal renal function and offer them prenatal therapy. However, the selection criteria remain as a problem. If actions are taken when the fetus is clearly at risk of fetal death, renal function is frequently already seriously impaired. To avoid this, fetal therapy should be done at an early stage, but then the question about whether or not the fetus needs the treatment is still unsolved.

After a local anaesthesia injection, a cannula with trochar is passed through the maternal abdominal wall and the uterus into the fetal bladder. The trochar is removed and a catheter is placed inside the cannula. The original catheter, a double J-stent, was soon modified into a double pigtail catheter. A short-length rod is used to push the end of the catheter into the fetal bladder and the longer one pushes the remaining catheter into the amniotic space. Some advances with the technique include the use of amnio-infusion prior to catheter insertion, antibiotic prophylaxis and the use of fetal paralysis. The improvements in ultrasound visualization have made the procedure easier. The most frequent complication is still shunt displacement which occurs in 19% of cases. Other complications include preterm labour (12%), chorio-amnionitis (5%) and procedure-related complications such as shunt obstruction, inadequate decompression of the fetal urinary tract or fetal injury during placement.[28]

An overall neonatal survival of 61% was reported using the procedure after adequate selection criteria;[29] an associated 4.8% of procedure-related loss rate has also been reported.[28]

An alternative to shunting not used in the UK for obstructive uropathy is open fetal surgery which requires hysterotomy and exteriorization of the fetus; this can lead to a high rate of complications. A third approach is percutaneous fetal

Clinical applications of fetal therapy

33

cystoscopy which has been used to confirm the ultrasonographic diagnosis of posterior urethral valves and to perform endoscopic fulguration of the valves.[30] Laser treatment may be useful to treat other causes of obstruction, such as some cases of urethrocele. A large, bulging or prolapsing urethrocele is a recognised, but rare, cause of bladder outlet obstruction. In these cases, a lack or delay of treatment may lead to bilateral renal damage. Options for treatment include placement of a vesico-amniotic shunt or cystoscopic-guided laser incision.[31] The latter can be done under ultrasound guidance minimizing the risks of the procedure.[32]

FETAL PLEURAL EFFUSIONS

Fetal chylothorax is associated with increased perinatal mortality. Intra-uterine management of the condition remains controversial because spontaneous resolution has been reported. Conservative treatment has been a satisfactory approach for small non-progressive effusions. However, the development of a mediastinal shift with significant lung compression, abnormal Doppler patterns in the great arteries before 35 weeks' gestation or hydrops are findings that indicate the need for prenatal treatment. This therapy aims to prolong pregnancy and prevent pulmonary hypoplasia and/or reversal of fetal hydrops. There are two major forms of treatment available for fetuses with chylothorax: thoracentesis and thoraco-amniotic shunting. Thoracentesis is a diagnostic procedure to obtain pleural fluid and establish whether or not the effusion is chylous; however, the principal drawback of therapeutic intervention is the rapid re-accumulation of effusion which usually occurs.[33] Pleuro-amniotic shunting provides a continuous decompression of the fetal chest, allowing lung expansion. In nearly half the cases, the placement of only one shunt permits a total regression of pleural effusion and a favourable outcome. In cases of isolated primary fetal pleural effusion, the survival rate of fetuses treated with thoraco-amniotic shunting is 92% compared to 50% in untreated cases.[34,35] Nevertheless, the procedure is not free of complications (shunt migration, obstruction, preterm labour, premature rupture of membranes, *etc.*) which may cause a poor outcome.

An intriguing non-invasive approach has been to use dietary manipulation. A low-fat, high medium-chain triglyceride maternal diet to reduce fetal lymphatic flow has been tried,[36] with the rationale of diminishing chyle production and flow. In neonates with chylothorax, triglycerides that persist on total parenteral nutrition and are, therefore, consistent with a non-enteral origin have been reported to contain 3-fold more long-chain unsaturated fatty acids of greater than or equal to 20 carbons (including 6-fold more arachidonic than the circulating serum triglycerides). Maternal feeding with medium-chain triglyceride diets could change the lymph composition in the fetus; however, the efficacy of this treatment needs to be confirmed.

FETAL DRUG THERAPY

Maternal administration of medication has been used to reach the fetus to treat several conditions. The best example is the administration of anti-arrhythmic agents to treat fetal supraventricular tachycardia arrhythmias. Digoxin is the drug most commonly used drug, but the effectiveness in hydropic fetuses seems poor. Other agents include sotalol or flecainide which both seem to be very effective.

Other examples include the use of corticosteroids to promote fetal lung maturation, to treat fetal heart block or congenital adrenal hyperplasia. Indomethacin has been tried to reduce fetal renal urine production and so idiopathic polyhydramnios.

If maternal–fetal transfer of the medication is not possible or not in sufficient quantities, direct fetal therapy has sometimes been tried. Intra-amniotic injection of thyroid hormones in cases of hypothyroid fetal goitre seems to be effective. Fetal intramuscular and intraperitoneal routes have also been used: in cases of arrhythmia, maternal administration is usually unsuccessful and intravenous fetal direct therapy has had a poor outcome.

OTHER PROCEDURES

AMNIO-INFUSION

There is evidence that amnio-infusion is associated with improvements in perinatal outcome when used for meconium-stained liquor in labour, particularly in hospitals where facilities for perinatal surveillance are limited.[37] The procedure seems to reduce the occurrence of variable decelerations and decrease Caesarean section, especially in settings where Caesarean sections are indicated based only on abnormal fetal heart rate alone and not in combination with fetal blood sampling.[38] However, the trials are too small to address the possibility of rare, but serious, maternal adverse effects of the procedure. A nasogastric tube is inserted transcervically into the uterine cavity just above the fetal presentation. Initially, 500 ml of normal saline (at room temperature) is infused through the tube over 30 min, and then a further 500 ml usually at a rate of 3 ml/min. There is no useful evidence concerning amnio-infusion to treat oligohydramnios for preterm rupture of membranes.[39]

SEALING OF MEMBRANES IN PRETERM PREMATURE RUPTURE OF MEMBRANES

Some cases of preterm premature rupture of membranes can be treated effectively with the intra-amniotic injection of platelets and cryoprecipitate. The technique does not require knowledge of the exact location of the defect, although isolated cases of unexpected fetal death related to the procedure have been reported. The appropriate dose of platelets and cryoprecipitate needs to be established.[40]

TRACHEAL OCCLUSION

Occlusion of the fetal trachea blocks the normal outflow of fetal lung fluid and stimulates the growth of hypoplastic lungs in fetuses with diaphragmatic hernia. Endoscopically-guided procedures may include a tracheal clip[41] or an inflatable balloon,[42] and prenatal tracheal occlusion can result in impressive lung growth in fetuses with severe congenital diaphragmatic hernia. However, survival remains compromised by pulmonary functional abnormality and the consequences of prematurity.[43]

TREATMENT FOR TUMOURS

The first successful resection of open surgery for fetal sacrococcygeal teratoma with long-term survival was reported by Adzick et al. in 1997.[44] There are only a few isolated cases reported in the literature. The main concerns are premature rupture of membranes, preterm delivery, and a high rate of fetal mortality. Less invasive interventions such as the use of laser to occlude selective feeding vessels of the tumours may be useful in the future.

EX UTERO INTRAPARTUM TREATMENT (EXIT PROCEDURE)

Ex utero intrapartum treatment (EXIT procedure) describes a procedure for maintaining fetal gas exchange until adequate ventilation is achieved when there is a potentially life-threatening airway obstruction at birth. The operation has been described in the treatment of giant fetal neck masses, such as lymphangiomas and cervical teratomas,[45] and in a case of laryngeal atresia. The reason for performing the procedure is that delay in adequately ventilating the neonate with airway obstruction can lead to hypoxia, acidosis, brain injury and death. The uteroplacental circulation is preserved by only partially delivering the fetus and maintaining uterine relaxation throughout the procedure. This requires a carefully co-ordinated, multidisciplinary treatment of a fetus at birth.

FUTURE POSSIBILITIES

STEM CELL TRANSPLANTATION

Some severe congenital problems, particularly haematological anomalies, may be treated by bone marrow transplantation. This procedure can be done postnatally, but the problems of rejection and graft versus host disease remain. Hopefully, fetal stem cells are able to proliferate, differentiate and become tolerant to host antigens so the disadvantages of the postnatal transplantation may be reduced. A correct and acute early prenatal diagnosis of the condition is essential for application of this procedure.

GENE THERAPY

Prenatal gene therapy may have an important place in the future. Some believe gene transfer and permanent integration of foreign DNA will be more effective in the developing fetus than in a child or adult.[46] Also it is hoped by doing this before the fetal immune system is completely developed, this may permit induction of immune tolerance against vector and the therapeutic gene. Finally, early prenatal gene therapy could reduce the early secondary consequences of the disease. Despite this, currently, prenatal gene therapy would be an option only if it is a life-threatening disease where prenatal therapy should have clear advantage over postnatal gene therapy. Pre-protocols for human prenatal gene therapy have been presented for treating α-thalassemia and a severe combined immunodeficiency disorder caused by deficiency of the adenosine deaminase enzyme due to mutations in the adenosine deaminase gene.[47]

Key points for clinical practice

- Fetal therapy is now more widely practiced and undergoing evidence-based evaluation. Early prenatal diagnosis and treatment in some clinical situations does offer benefits.

- Intra-uterine transfusion therapy has significantly improved the outcome of allo-immune disorders in pregnancy and human parvo-virus B19 infection.

- Several treatments have been introduced to treat twin-to-twin transfusion syndrome. While amniodrainage remains as a major therapeutic option, laser treatment seems to improve the outcomes further, particularly in early-onset cases, and may reduce neurological sequelae in the survivors when one of the twins dies.

- Shunting procedures are useful in cases of fetal lower urinary tract obstruction by preventing pulmonary hypoplasia and neonatal death, and preserving renal function in some cases. In pleural effusions, especially from chylothorax, pleuro-amniotic shunting is a valuable procedure to prevent or treat fetal hydrops and death.

- In cases of fetal arrhythmias, administration of maternal anti-arrhythmic agents such as digoxin or, more recently, flecainide may resolve this dangerous situation. In unsuccessful cases, direct fetal therapy can be considered.

- There is a wide variety of other procedures with prospects for the future such as stem cell transplantation or gene therapy.

References

1. Liley AW. Intrauterine transfusion of foetus in haemolytic disease. *BMJ* 1963; **2**: 1107–1109.
2. Rodeck CH, Kemp JR, Holman CA, Whitmore CA, Karnicki J, Austin MA. Direct intravascular fetal blood transfusion by fetoscopy in severe Rhesus isoimmunisation. *Lancet* 1981; **I**: 625–627.
3. Bang J, Bock JE, Trolle D. Ultrasound-guided fetal intravenous transfusion for severe rhesus haemolytic disease. *BMJ* 1982; **284**: 373–374.
4. Abdel-Fattah SA, Soothill PW, Carroll SG, Kyle PM. Non-invasive diagnosis of anemia in hydrops fetalis with the use of middle cerebral artery Doppler velocity. *Am J Obstet Gynecol* 2001; **185**: 1411–1415.
5. Gonsoulin WJ, Moise Jr KJ, Milam JD, Sala JD, Weber VW, Carpenter Jr RJ. Serial maternal blood donations for intrauterine transfusion. *Obstet Gynecol* 1990; **75**: 158–162.
6. Shumacher B, Moise Jr KJ. Fetal transfusion for red blood cell alloimmunization in pregnancy. *Obstet Gynecol* 1996; **88**: 137–150.
7. Queenan JT. Rh-disease: a perinatal success story. *Obstet Gynecol* 2002; **100**: 405–406.
8. Soothill P. Intrauterine blood transfusion for non-immune hydrops fetalis due to parvovirus B19 infection. *Lancet* 1990; **336**: 121–122.
9. Sharif U, Kuban K. Prenatal intracranial hemorrhage and neurologic complications in alloimmune thrombocytopenia. *J Child Neurol* 2001; **16**: 838–842.
10. Overton TG, Duncan KR, Jolly M, Letsky E, Fisk NM. Serial aggressive platelet transfusion for fetal alloimmune thrombocytopenia: platelet dynamics and perinatal outcome. *Am J Obstet Gynecol* 2002; **186**: 826–831.
11. Spencer JA, Burrows RF. Feto-maternal alloimmune thrombocytopenia: a literature review and statistical analysis. *Aust NZ J Obstet Gynaecol* 2001; **41**: 45–55.

12. Murphy MF, Rayment R, Allen D, Roberts D. fetal and neonatal treatment for alloimmune thrombocytopenia. In: Hadley A, Soothill PW. (eds) *Alloimmune Disorders of Pregnancy*. Cambridge: Cambridge University Press, 2002; 253–278.

13. Roberts D, Neilson JP, Weindling AM. Interventions for the treatment of twin-to-twin transfusion syndrome. *Cochrane Database Syst Rev* 2001; **1**: CD002073.

14. Abdel-Fattah SA, Carroll SG, Kyle PM, Soothill PW. Amniodrainage: how much to drain? *Fetal Diagn Ther* 1999; **14**: 279–282.

15. Pinette MG, Pan Y, Pinette SG, Stubblefield PG. Treatment of twin-twin transfusion syndrome. *Obstet Gynecol* 1993; **82**: 841–846.

16. Jauniaux E, Holmes A, Hyett J, Yates R, Rodeck C. Rapid and radical amniodrainage in the treatment of severe twin-twin transfusion syndrome. *Prenat Diagn* 2001; **21**: 471–476.

17. DeLia JE, Cruikshank DP, Keye WR. Fetoscopic neodymium:YAG laser occlusion of placental vessels in severe twin-twin transfusion syndrome. *Obstet Gynecol* 1990; **75**: 1046–1053.

18. Ville Y, Hyett J, Hecher K, Nicolaides KH. Preliminary experience with endoscopic laser surgery for severe twin-twin transfusion syndrome. *N Engl J Med* 1995; **332**: 224–227.

19. De Lia JE, Kuhlmann RS, Harstad TW, Cruikshank DP. Fetoscopic laser ablation of placental vessels in severe previable twin-twin transfusion syndrome. *Am J Obstet Gynecol* 1995; **172**: 1202–1211.

20. Denbow ML, Cox P, Taylor M, Hammal DM, Fisk NM. Placental angioarchitecture in monochorionic twin pregnancies: relationship to fetal growth, fetofetal transfusion syndrome, and pregnancy outcome. *Am J Obstet Gynecol* 2000; **182**: 417–426.

21. Saade GR, Belfort MA, Berry DL *et al*. Amniotic septostomy for the treatment of twin oligohydramnios-polyhydramnios sequence. *Fetal Diagn Ther* 1998; **13**: 86–93.

22. Johnson JR, Rossi KQ, O'Shaughnessy RW. Amnioreduction versus septostomy in twin-twin transfusion syndrome. *Am J Obstet Gynecol* 2001; **185**: 1044–1047.

23. Soothill P, Sohan K, Carroll S, Kyle P. Ultrasound-guided, intra-abdominal laser to treat acardiac pregnancies. *Br J Obstet Gynaecol* 2002; **109**: 352–354.

24. Taylor MJ, Shalev E, Tanawattanacharoen S *et al*. Ultrasound-guided umbilical cord occlusion using bipolar diathermy for stage III/IV twin-twin transfusion syndrome. *Prenat Diagn* 2002; **22**: 70–76.

25. Manning FA, Harrison MR, Rodeck C. Catheter shunts for fetal hydronephrosis and hydrocephalus. Report of the International Fetal Surgery Registry. *N Engl J Med* 1986; **315**: 336–340.

26. Freedman AL, Johnson MP, Gonzalez R. Fetal therapy for obstructive uropathy: past, present...future? *Pediatr Nephrol* 2000; **14**: 167–176

27. Crombleholme TM, Harrison MR, Golbus MS *et al*. Fetal intervention in obstructive uropathy: prognostic indicators and efficacy of intervention. *Am J Obstet Gynecol* 1990; **162**: 1239–1244.

28. Elder JS, Duckett Jr JW, Synder HM. Intervention for fetal obstructive uropathy: has it been effective? *Lancet* 1987; **II**: 1007–1010.

29. Freedman AL, Bukowski TP, Smith CA, Evans MI, Johnson MP, Gonzalez R. Fetal therapy for obstructive uropathy: diagnosis specific outcomes. *J Urol* 1996; **156**: 720–724.

30. Quintero RA, Hume R, Smith C *et al*. Percutaneous fetal cystoscopy and endoscopic fulguration of posterior urethral valves. *Am J Obstet Gynecol* 1995; **172**: 206–209.

31. Quintero RA, Homsy Y, Bornick PW, Allen M, Johnson PK. *In utero* treatment of fetal bladder-outlet obstruction by a urethrocele. *Lancet* 2001; **357**: 1947–1948.

32. Soothill PW, Bartha JL, Tizard J. Ultrasound-guided laser treatment for fetal bladder outlet obstruction secondary to urethrocele. *Am J Obstet Gynecol* 2002; In press.

33. Aubard Y, Derouineau I, Aubard V, Chalifour V, Preux PM. Primary fetal hydrothorax: a literature review and proposed antenatal clinical strategy. *Fetal Diagn Ther* 1998; **13**: 325–333.

34. Nicolaides KH, Azar GB. Thoraco-amniotic shunting. *Fetal Diagn Ther* 1990; **5**: 153–164.

35. Hagay Z, Reece A, Roberts A, Hobbins JC. Isolated fetal pleural effusion: a prenatal management dilemma. *Obstet Gynecol* 1993; **81**: 147–152.

36. Bartha JL, Comino-Delgado R. Fetal chylothorax response to maternal dietary treatment. *Obstet Gynecol* 2001; **97**: 820–823.

37. Hofmeyr GJ. Amnioinfusion for meconium-stained liquor in labour. *Cochrane Database Syst Rev* 2002; **1**: CD000014.

38. Hofmeyr GJ. Amnioinfusion for umbilical cord compression in labour. *Cochrane Database Syst Rev* 2000; **2**: CD000013.

39. Hofmeyr GJ. Amnioinfusion for preterm rupture of membranes. *Cochrane Database Syst Rev* 2000; **2**: CD000942.

40. Quintero RA, Morales WJ, Allen M, Bornick PW, Arroyo J, LeParc G. Treatment of iatrogenic previable premature rupture of membranes with intra-amniotic injection of platelets and cryoprecipitate (amniopatch): preliminary experience. *Am J Obstet Gynecol* 1999; **181**: 744–749.

41. VanderWall KJ, Bruch SW, Meuli M *et al*. Fetal endoscopic ('Fetendo') tracheal clip. *J Pediatr Surg* 1996; **31**: 1101–1103.

42. Deprest JA, Evrard VA, Van Ballaer PP *et al*. Tracheoscopic endoluminal plugging using an inflatable device in the fetal lamb model. *Eur J Obstet Gynecol Reprod Biol* 1998; **81**: 165–169.

43. Flake AW, Crombleholme TM, Johnson MP, Howell LJ, Adzick NS. Treatment of severe congenital diaphragmatic hernia by fetal tracheal occlusion: clinical experience with fifteen cases. *Am J Obstet Gynecol* 2000; **183**: 1059–1066.

44. Adzick NS, Crombleholme TM, Morgan MA, Quinn TM. A rapidly growing fetal teratoma. *Lancet* 1997; **349**: 538.

45. Murphy DJ, Kyle PM, Cairns P, Weir P, Cusick E, Soothill PW. *Ex utero* intrapartum treatment for cervical teratoma. *Br J Obstet Gynaecol* 2001; **108**: 429–430.

46. Zanjan ED, Anderson WF. Prospects for *in utero* human gene therapy. *Science* 1999; **285**: 2084–2088.

47. Staff AC. An introduction to gene therapy and its potential prenatal use. *Acta Obstet Gynecol Scand* 2001; **80**: 485–491.

Stephen A. Walkinshaw Lindsay Cochrane

4

Investigation and management of the small fetus

A fetus is said to be small for gestational age if it falls below defined measurements determined by centiles or standard deviations from the mean for a normal population. Definitions vary both in the measurement used, abdominal circumference or estimated fetal weight by various formulae, and by the centile used, 2.5th, 3rd, 5th, 10th, 15th, and 25th. The most commonly used definition of small for gestational age is below the 10th centile for abdominal circumference or estimated fetal weight. Some have argued that both abdominal circumference and estimated weight should be less than the chosen centile before labelling an individual fetus small.

The small baby is vulnerable, not only to death or damage that may be inflicted by inadequate intra-uterine nutrition, but also to the complications of prematurity which may occur iatrogenically. At present, little can be done to treat fetal growth restriction (FGR) and so, in most cases, the only intervention open to the obstetrician is to deliver the baby prematurely. A number of investigations of fetal behaviour and placental function are used to guide timing of delivery, but a great degree of uncertainty exists, both between clinicians in a similar situation and in an individual clinician facing different clinical situations.[1]

Having identified that a fetus is small for gestational age, the challenge to the clinician is to: (i) determine whether the fetus is reaching its growth potential or is growth-restricted; (ii) identify any underlying cause and monitor appropriately; and (iii) deliver at the optimum time so as to minimise the damage to the baby both from intra-uterine factors and from prematurity.

Stephen A. Walkinshaw BSc MD MRCOG, Consultant in Maternal and Fetal Medicine, Liverpool Women's Hospital, Crown Street, Liverpool L8 7SS, UK (for correspondence)

Lindsay Cochrane MB ChB MRCOG, Specialist Registrar, Liverpool Women's Hospital, Crown Street, Liverpool L8 7SS, UK

WHAT ARE WE WORRIED ABOUT?

STILLBIRTH

A fetus that is small for gestational age is at a 15-fold increased risk of intra-uterine fetal death compared to an appropriately grown fetus.[2]. In so-called 'unexplained' stillbirths, 20% show evidence of FGR. In the *8th Annual CESDI Report*, reviewing unexplained stillbirths from 1996–1997, 14% of the comments on substandard care related to FGR. There was criticism not only of failure to pick up small babies, but also of inadequate monitoring or action taken in those babies known to be small. The panel commented on the lack of evidence and consensus about the best screening and monitoring tools for FGR.

INTRAPARTUM HYPOXIA

Caesarean section for fetal distress is increased and there are low 5-min Apgar scores, severe acidaemia at delivery and neonatal resuscitation requiring intubation in small for gestational age compared to appropriate for gestational age infants.[3]

NEONATAL COMPLICATIONS

Neonatal morbidity and mortality are increased in small for gestational age babies and more marked in those with the lowest birth-weights. Neonatal mortality is increased in small for gestational age infants born at any gestational age; for example, at 38 weeks' gestation, the neonatal mortality for small for gestational age babies is 1%, compared with 0.2% for appropriately grown infants.

In preterm small for gestational age infants, respiratory distress requiring ventilation and grade 3 and 4 intraventricular haemorrhage are increased as compared with appropriate for gestational age infants of the same gestational period. In term small for gestational age infants, seizures in the first 24 h of life and neonatal sepsis are increased.[3]

IMPAIRED NEURODEVELOPMENT

Small for gestational age, very preterm infants (less than 32 weeks' gestation) are more likely to have long-term neuromotor dysfunction than appropriate for gestational age babies of the same gestation. The type of dysfunction appears to be specific for small for gestational age infants, with gross motor dysfunction and minor neurological dysfunction being prominent, rather than cerebral palsy, which is more common in appropriate for gestational age preterm babies. There is an increased need for special education at aged 9 years with only 34% of small for gestational age, very preterm infants able to follow mainstream education compared to 46% of appropriate for gestational age children.

Term infants born small for gestational age demonstrate deficits in academic achievement. They are less likely to be in the top 15% of academic achievement and are more likely to require special education than those born appropriate for gestational age (5% *versus* 2%). Poor school performance is increased with a reduction in birth-weight centile.

In adult life, those born small for gestational age were less likely to have professional or managerial jobs and had significantly lower incomes than those born appropriate for gestational age. These differences were still present following adjustment for other factors including social class.[4]

COMPLICATIONS IN ADULT LIFE

In addition to the more immediate effects of being born small for gestational age, evidence is now emerging of an increased incidence of problems in later life, specifically obesity, non-insulin dependent diabetes, hypertension and cardiovascular disease. This has been confirmed in a number of different populations world-wide.[5]

DIAGNOSIS OF THE SMALL BABY

IDENTIFYING SMALL FOR GESTATIONAL AGE FETUSES

A potential small fetus may come to the attention of clinicians through different routes. The low-risk population is 'screened' by clinical estimates of fetal size, either subjective or by symphyseal fundal height measurement. The reported sensitivities and specificities of these methods vary widely with abdominal palpation alone having a sensitivity of around 30%, symphyseal fundal height having reported sensitivities of 27–86% and specificity of around 80%. Only one randomised-controlled trial of these two methods has been carried out, and did not show any difference in perinatal outcome between the two groups.[6]

Third trimester ultrasound has not been shown to improve outcome when applied routinely to a whole population in late pregnancy. Targeted screening may identify other pregnancies by ultrasound where there is a perceived risk of growth restriction.

CHECK THE GESTATIONAL AGE

Accurate determination of the gestation is essential to identify that a fetus is small for gestational age. Ultrasound scan has been shown to improve the accuracy of dating in large populations, with first trimester ultrasound the most useful. However, a second trimester scan may also provide useful dating information.

USE THE CORRECT MEASUREMENTS

Abdominal circumference has the highest sensitivity and estimated fetal weight the highest odds ratio for detecting small for gestational age at birth.[7] Several formulae are available to estimate fetal weight using abdominal circumference alone (Campbell) or with the addition of biparietal diameter (Shepherd) and/or femur length (Aoki/Hadlock, respectively). Comparative studies of various formulae have been undertaken. In general, most formulae perform best at the smaller weights, but in practical terms there is little between the various formulae. Clinicians should be aware of the magnitude and direction of the systematic error for the formula they use, and the inherent size of the general error in ultrasound estimated weights. Most tend to underestimate compared to actual weight at birth. There is some evidence that abdominal circumference is more accurately measured using an ellipse than the trace method. Measurements must be plotted on the correct chart. The chart must be derived from data on a similar population measuring the same dimensions in the same way as was used in compilation of the chart. It is more appropriate for a single measurement to assess fetal size to be plotted on a chart derived from cross-sectional data.

A newer development is the use of customised growth-charts. These allow adjustment for maternal height, weight, parity, ethnic origin, and for fetal sex, giving an individual growth-chart for each patient. This can reduce the number of false positives and contribute towards the distinction between constitutionally small and growth-restricted babies.[8] The use of customised growth-charts has been shown to reduce the proportion of babies with a normal outcome diagnosed as small for gestational age at any point during serial growth scans. Customised charts may be generated from a computer model using software available free on the internet (<www.gestation.net>).

DETERMINING RISK

The important question is whether the fetus is pathologically growth restricted, has an abnormality or is small but healthy. A number of factors are taken into consideration when assessing the risk to the fetus.

RISK FACTORS

When reviewing an ultrasound report that suggests a small for gestation fetus, the first question is: does the history point to a likely growth-restricted fetus? Factors in a woman's history that will increase the chances of a growth-restricted baby include: (i) previous history of FGR; (ii) medical disorders (such as hypertension or connective tissue disorder); (iii) drugs (such as amphetamines or cigarette smoking); and (iv) poor nutrition or adverse socio-economic factors. Issues identified during pregnancy may increase the chances of FGR: examples include early pregnancy bleeding, antepartum haemorrhage, maternal pre-eclampsia, echogenic fetal bowel or unexplained raised maternal serum α-fetoprotein.

At present, ultrasound screening for small for gestational age is not practised, but many areas use uterine artery Doppler velocimetry to identify pregnancies at risk. There is debate on the efficacy of this approach, and on the precise index or measurement,[9] but in a low-risk population, a woman with a positive uterine artery Doppler test has a likelihood ratio of 3.6 for developing small for gestational age (95% CI, 2.3–3.4). Conversely, where the test is negative, the likelihood ratio is 0.8 (95% CI, 0.8–0.9).

TIME OF ONSET

Early detection of a small for gestation fetus is more likely to be associated with true growth restriction, fetal abnormality, or infection. Some studies have suggested that 5–40% of growth-restricted fetuses before 32 weeks' gestation have evidence of congenital infection. At earlier gestation, particularly in the absence of other risk factors or co-existing hypertensive disease, the risk of chromosomal abnormality may be as high as 20%.

FETAL SIZE

The smaller the fetus, the greater the chance of true growth restriction. Perinatal mortality and morbidity is higher in those with the greatest degree of growth retardation. The risk of a chromosome abnormality is also higher in the most severely growth-restricted.

FETAL ANOMALIES

Where the fetus has measured small, a full anatomical survey should be repeated in view of the increased incidence of fetal anomaly amongst small for gestational age babies. If a structural abnormality has been identified, this may explain fetal size

UMBILICAL ARTERY DOPPLER

Good laboratory evidence indicates that where growth restriction is secondary to placental vascular damage blood velocity measurements in the umbilical artery become abnormal. The type of histological vessel change and the precise mechanisms of blood velocity change are still debated, and may be more complex than initially suspected.[10]

A number of different measurements are used to describe the relationship between systolic and diastolic flow in the umbilical artery. All of these show good reproducibility and correlation with outcome. Resistance index is the difference between peak systolic and end diastolic frequency divided by peak systolic frequency. A study comparing resistance index with pulsatility index, S/D ratio and diastolic-average ratio has shown resistance index to be the most discriminatory for predicting poor outcome.[11]

European and Australian studies[12,13] have clearly demonstrated the relationship between both mortality and morbidity with increasing severity of Doppler index. This relationship applied across all gestations.

Measurement of the umbilical artery waveform is, therefore, the most important discriminator in the small for gestational age infant. This is widely used, relatively easy to perform, and allows identification of the fetus likely to be growth restricted because of placental dysfunction. The test has an excellent negative predictive value for perinatal mortality and morbidity, but its positive predictive value is relatively low.[14] Normal umbilical artery Doppler can be regarded as re-assuring, and is associated with a low risk of perinatal mortality. Debate continues on whether such pregnancies are at similar risk to appropriately grown fetuses. Most studies still show excess morbidity in infants that are small with normal Doppler compared with normally grown infants. This is particularly true where infants are less than the third centile.

AMNIOTIC FLUID VOLUME

Ultrasonic assessment of amniotic fluid is frequently used as part of the assessment of the small fetus. Reduced liquor volume, however measured, has been recognised for many years as associated with small for gestation fetuses that are growth restricted. Increased abnormal outcomes, including mortality, have been demonstrated with decreasing liquor volumes, particularly where pool depths of less than 2 cm are found.[15] Changes in liquor volume are generally thought to occur late in the sequence of fetal adaptation to poor growth, but in one study of small for gestational age fetuses, a reduced amniotic fluid index was been found early in the progression of FGR, at a similar stage to abnormal umbilical artery Doppler.[16] Amniotic fluid volume has a good negative predictive value for poor outcome (98%) in the small for gestational age fetus and so is re-assuring when normal.

Increased liquor volume is an unusual finding where the fetus is measured small and should raise strong suspicion of fetal abnormality, particularly syndromal associations. Sickler *et al.*[17] showed that over 90% of fetuses with estimated weights less than the 10th centile and hydramnios had major malformations at birth, and in one-quarter of cases antenatal detection was not possible. Over one-third had chromosomal anomalies.

Controversy remains over the measurement of liquor volume and the definition of reduced liquor volume. Amniotic fluid index appears to reflect measured amniotic fluid volume better than maximum pool depth, but clinical studies have not been able to demonstrate advantage and may lead to an over diagnosis of oligohydramnios and hydramnios. A number of reference ranges are available, derived from different populations and using different methodologies. The recent publication of the tables and charts of Magann *et al.*[18] should resolve this debate, as these were derived using robust methods. Liquor volume estimates should always be related to gestational age.

FURTHER INVESTIGATIONS

INVASIVE TESTING

Up to 19% of severely growth-restricted babies will have chromosome abnormalities. The decision to carry out an invasive test can be difficult. Clearly, if structural abnormalities are present, it would be appropriate to offer karyotyping. Infants that are extremely small may justify consideration of invasive testing. The presence of increased liquor or growth restriction of early onset with no predisposing factors should routinely lead to an offer of invasive testing. Rapid techniques may not necessarily be appropriate, as structural re-arrangements may be present. Consideration should be given to techniques to detect some of the microdeletion abnormalities, and consultation with the genetic laboratories may be needed. A number of studies have reported high rates of chromosome and structural abnormalities in fetuses with abnormal umbilical artery Doppler. The best rule is that where the features do not clearly fit a pattern, then consider invasive tests. A screen for congenital infection in small for gestational age babies should be part of the investigation.

GROWTH VELOCITY

The most likely result of the preliminary assessment will be to ask for another scan. Growth velocity is an important part of monitoring the small for gestational age infant where immediate delivery is not considered necessary from the primary investigations. Serial measurements of abdominal circumference or estimated fetal weight are better for demonstrating growth restriction than a single measurement, which can only determine whether or not a fetus is small for gestational age at a particular point. Due to the known inter- and intra-observer error in measurement, it is usually recommended that measurements are not repeated more frequently than every 2 weeks.

Charts in common use are derived from cross-sectional data and, in theory, these should not be used to plot serial measures. Growth velocity can be inferred from knowledge of the average expected growth of the key parameters of abdominal circumference. The mean abdominal circumference growth each week is approximately 10 mm. A number of authors have estimated the average fetal weight gain per week at different gestational ages, and these data can be used to judge growth velocity without the need for charting.

Charts are available from longitudinally derived data and these may be more appropriate for assessing growth velocity in an individual fetus.[19] The statistical algorithms used for these charts are difficult, and many find them too complex for routine use. The use of z-scores, that is determining the estimated fetal weight in terms of standard deviations from the mean, may also improve accuracy in assessing growth velocity rather than just assessing the growth velocity visually against defined centile growth lines. For example, if estimated fetal weight is calculated as 1.9 SD below the mean at initial measurement and 1.9 at the next, this growth is known to be adequate without having to chart and visually assess the growth.

WHEN TO DELIVER

As has been shown above, a number of factors are associated with perinatal mortality and morbidity in the small for gestational age fetus. However, the strongest determinant of postnatal outcome remains gestational age at delivery.[15] Timing of delivery is complex because it requires balancing the risks of continuing intra-uterine life, death or damage due to hypoxaemia, against the risks of prematurity. The aim in the very preterm fetus is to allow the pregnancy to continue to the point just before damage occurs. To allow this decision, an assessment of fetal health has to be carried out, and there needs to be an understanding of the predictive value of the use of these assessments to time delivery.

UMBILICAL DOPPLER

Systematic review and meta-analyses of randomised controlled trials using umbilical artery Doppler, involving a total of over 7000 patients,[20] shows that the use of umbilical artery Doppler causes a statistically significant reduction in perinatal mortality (odds ratio 0.62; 95% CI, 0.45–0.85). A later meta-analysis by the same authors excluded one study about which there later became some doubt.[21] This still showed a significant trend towards reduced perinatal mortality, but just failed to reach statistical significance (odd ratio 0.81; 95% CI, 0.5–1.01). Both meta-analyses showed a significant reduction in antenatal admissions, induction of labour and emergency Caesarean section for fetal distress with no adverse effects found, although the overall rate of Caesarean section was unchanged. Doppler imaging may improve outcome by targeting induction and elective Caesarean delivery more appropriately.

In most of the studies looking at the effect of umbilical artery Doppler in high-risk pregnancy, there was no standardised management protocol based on the Doppler results. The information from Doppler investigation was made available to clinicians when their patient was in the intervention group, but they made their own decisions about management based on all the available clinical information. The review tells us that knowledge of the Doppler result improves outcome, but not the basis on which clinicians timed individual deliveries.

As part of the process of devising the GRIT Trial,[1] 49 European obstetricians were asked when they would advise delivery in a growth-restricted baby given different gestational ages with a range of Doppler waveforms and CTG variability measures. Their responses showed disagreement and uncertainty about when to deliver. Over half the obstetricians would recommend delivery in the presence of reversed EDF beyond 29 weeks' gestation, absent EDF beyond 32 weeks and severely reduced EDF beyond 35 weeks. Similarly, over half would delay delivery with severely reduced EDF below 31 weeks, absent EDF below 28 weeks and reversed EDF below 25 weeks. Between these areas was a band of collective uncertainty.

The growth restriction intervention trial (GRIT), which is due to report soon, addresses this issue of timing. The evidence available, so far, from the trial is that early delivery appears to offer no advantage for immediate outcomes.

Serial umbilical Doppler measures are common practice, though the evidence base is scanty. Given the knowledge of the relationship between particular patterns and outcomes, detection of the timing of the appearance of either absent or reversed velocities is important and will influence care. The ideal frequency of examination is not known. Where indices are abnormal but there are forward velocities, there is less information from serial measures. Some data suggest that if these remain static or improve, the outcomes approach those of a normal Doppler group; where values rise, then outcomes can be as poor as those for absent velocities. There are no longitudinal charts, and great care is needed if values are plotted on cross sectional charts.

TESTS OF FETAL WELL-BEING

The key is to avoid or to detect as early as possible fetal hypoxaemia or acidosis. CTG is widely used for antenatal assessment of the fetus in a number of circumstances including the small for gestational age fetus. Observational data have shown abnormal CTG, with reduced variability or decelerations, to be associated with an increase in perinatal mortality and morbidity. Computerised CTGs appear more accurate in predicting poor outcome than subjective assessment. Animal work clarified some of the relationships between fetal acid-base balance and fetal heart rate changes. Work examining antenatal blood gas analysis by cordocentesis has shown a relationship between fetal pO_2 and short-term variability particularly using computerised CTG analysis. Others have shown threshold values for antenatal acid-base values, below which CTG changes tend to occur.

In spite of the biological relationships, meta-analysis of the use of conventional CTGs in high- and medium-risk pregnancy has shown no evidence of benefit. In fact, there was a trend towards increased perinatal mortality in the CTG monitored group.[22] Evidence from neurodevelopmental studies in the 1980s suggested that small for gestational age infants with abnormal cardiotocography did poorly compared with infants of similar size who had normal heart rate patterns. This may suggest that waiting until obvious changes occur may be too late.

The BPP is a fetal assessment that was based on the Apgar score, incorporating measures of tone, movement, breathing and heart rate (using CTG) but using amniotic fluid volume as an indirect measure of renal blood flow. There is an association between chronic fetal compromise and decreased fetal body and breathing movements, changes in the CTG and oligohydramnios. Sheep models have elucidated the sequence of change in biophysical parameters and the degree of fetal hypoxaemia, and observational studies have shown that there is a relationship between low BPP score and poor pregnancy outcome. Prospective studies in small for gestation fetuses have not demonstrated benefit over simpler monitoring techniques,[23] and a Cochrane Review of the subject showed no impact from the use of the BPP compared with the CTG alone

MIDDLE CEREBRAL ARTERY DOPPLER

A number of cardiovascular adaptations occur in the growth-restricted fetus. An increase in cerebral blood flow velocity, which is associated with a reduced pulsatility index or an increased cerebral to umbilical artery ratio, is seen in a large proportion of growth-restricted fetuses with abnormal umbilical artery Doppler. This has been seen as a 'brain sparing' effect whereby blood is redistributed in hypoxic fetuses so as to increase the cerebral circulation. Antenatal fetal blood sampling has shown a relationship between cerebral indices and hypoxaemia and acidosis. These fetuses are at increased risk of fetal distress in labour and admission to neonatal intensive care.[24,25] However, the term 'brain sparing' does seem to be accurate with no evidence of increased neurological impairment at aged 3 years.[26] In severe hypoxaemia, signs of fetal brain sparing have been seen to disappear terminally and so a single measurement may give false re-assurance in those most severely affected. Measuring the actual middle cerebral peak velocity rather than the pulsatility index may be more accurate in these fetuses.[14]

VENOUS DOPPLER

Observations of abnormalities of cardiac function and output in severely hypoxic, growth-restricted fetuses led to examination of the right heart and venous system for relationships between measures of blood flow, fetal acid-base balance and perinatal outcome. In growth-restricted fetuses, characteristic patterns of reversal of flow in the inferior vena cava and ductus venosus and pulsations in the umbilical vein have been observed at the end of diastole. These abnormal pulsations occur synchronously with atrial contraction and are thought to represent transmission of atrial contractions into the venous circulation. These abnormal venous waveforms are significantly associated with deteriorating acid-base status and poor perinatal outcome, they usually occur late and their association is stronger than that observed with arterial Doppler changes.[27,28]

The strongest association with poor outcome in small for gestational age below the 5th centile occurs with abnormal pulsations of the ductus venosus.[22,23] These are significantly associated with perinatal death; in one study, they had a positive predictive value of 80% and a negative predictive value of 93% for perinatal death.[18] These data suggest their occurrence is a late finding with a high incidence of fetal or neonatal death; therefore, delivery, once they have been identified may be too late to improve outcome. Other studies, while consistently showing abnormal ductus venosus Doppler to be a late finding and a poor prognostic sign, have not shown such an inevitable association with perinatal death.[16]

Umbilical venous Doppler has also been studied in fetuses with absent or reversed end diastolic flow in the umbilical artery. Their presence in a fetus with abnormal umbilical artery Doppler also appears to be a poor prognostic sign and indicate chronic intra-uterine hypoxaemia with a very poor perinatal outcome.[25] However, they occur more frequently than ductus venosus pulsations and their positive predictive vale for perinatal death is not so strong (36%, with a negative predictive value of 88%). This may, however, make their appearance more useful in timing intervention before perinatal death is inevitable.[14]

Prospective studies have shown that changes in venous waveforms predate changes in CTG parameters. The precise magnitude of the delay has varied, but it has generally been measured in days. This may offer an interventional window, but the use of venous Doppler has yet to be subjected to a randomised clinical trial.

Regardless of the gestation, there seems to be an order in which variables become abnormal in the growth-restricted fetus. Amniotic fluid index and umbilical artery Doppler are the first to become abnormal, followed by the middle cerebral artery, then by changes in the venous Doppler which occur at approximately the same time as a reduction in short-term variability on CTG. The poorest outcome appears to occur in those fetuses where both reduced short-term variability on CTG and abnormal ductus venosus Doppler occur together.[16] Deterioration in biophysical profile with a reduction in tone and movement occurs, in the majority, after Doppler deterioration is complete.[15]

Deterioration is not inevitable and, when it occurs, does so over a variable time-scale. Multivessel Doppler surveillance coupled with observation of short-term fetal heart rate variability has great potential for assessment of this type of small for gestational age fetus. However, their influence on outcome when used in clinical practice has yet to be evaluated.

THE PARENTS

Concern over a small fetus can be intense, particularly where diagnosis is early. Parents need to be kept informed of the likely diagnoses, the types of tests to be performed and their uncertainties, and the reasons why delivery might be necessary. If early delivery is being considered, they should meet with neonatal physicians. Realistic estimates of outcome, and the uncertainties of long-term follow-up should be honestly discussed. The use of neonatal gestation and weight-specific survival charts may be useful in deciding on timing of delivery and counselling parents.

THERAPY

At present, there are few treatment options other than delivery. Bed rest has been recommended, with some evidence of improved placental blood flow, but no clinical benefit has ever been demonstrated. Studies with low-dose aspirin have been carried out, but no benefit has been demonstrated in studies where aspirin has been started after the diagnosis of growth restriction. The finding that stress can alter uterine artery haemodynamics opens an interesting potential group of therapies.

As the main concern is the effect of fetal hypoxaemia on survival and long-term outcome, Nicolaides' group have examined the effects of maternal hyperoxygenation on the severely growth-restricted fetus. Changes in blood gas parameters occur, though in a larger study using aortic Doppler indices as a surrogate for hypoxia, it was clear that not all fetuses respond.[29] Three, small, randomised studies have examined the effects on perinatal survival of continuous maternal hyperoxygenation in severely growth-restricted infants with abnormal umbilical Doppler. All have shown a reduced perinatal mortality, although the two earlier trials have serious methodological flaws. The most recent study randomised small fetuses with absent umbilical artery end diastolic velocities at 24–30 weeks' gestation, and this would reflect a group with uncertainty about timing of delivery.[32] Overall survival in the three trials was 67% in the treated arms and 36% in the untreated arms. Interpretation of the results of small trials is always difficult, and no long-term data are available, but the intervention suggests promise in a specific group of growth-restricted fetuses.

STREAMLINING THE MANAGEMENT

A pragmatic scheme of management for the small for gestational age infant is shown in Figure 1, using a primary screen of assessment of fetal size, liquor volume and umbilical artery Doppler as a starting point. All should have had a full repeat anatomical survey, and considered to be normal. If liquor volume is increased, these fetuses should be managed as fetuses with a probable abnormality.

GROUP A

Small for gestational age and all indices normal:

- In the absence of risk factors and where EFW 3rd to 10th centile, re-scan in 4 weeks to check growth velocity.
- If risk factors and EFW 3rd to 10th centile, re-scan in 3 weeks.
- If EFW less than 3rd centile perform detailed scan, consider karyotype and congenital infection screen; re-scan in 3 weeks.

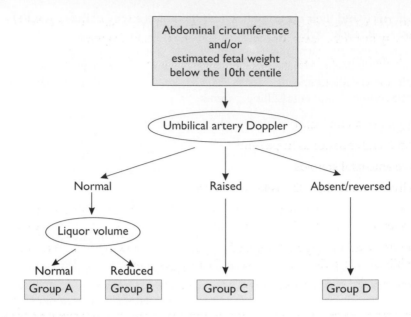

Fig. 1 Scheme of management for the small for gestational age infant.

At the next scan:

- If growth velocity and other indices are normal, no further follow-up is required.
- If indices are normal but growth velocity is reduced, again consider karyotype and infection screen.
- Use Z score or abdominal circumference 10 mm per week rule to determine velocity.
- If growth velocity is reduced and Dopplers or liquor volume are reduced, transfer to groups B, C or D.

GROUP B

Small for gestational age with normal Doppler but reduced liquor volume:

- If more than 37 weeks' gestation, consider delivery.
- If less than 37 weeks' gestation, repeat scan in 3 weeks and manage as for group A following the next scan.

GROUP C

Small for gestational age with reduced EDF:

- Repeat growth scan in 2 weeks.
- Repeat Doppler weekly.
- Taking gestational age and other risk factors into account, consider CTG or BPP monitoring. Monitoring should be no more frequent than twice weekly unless EFW/abdominal circumference less than 3rd centile.

- Consider delivery if greater than 36 weeks with evidence of poor growth velocity or further deterioration in the uterine artery Doppler.
- Give antenatal steroids if delivery less than 36 weeks' gestation.

GROUP D

Small for gestational age and absent or reversed EDF:

- Admit and monitor as in-patient.
- Give antenatal steroids.
- Deliver if more than 32 weeks' gestation.
- Monitor with daily or twice daily CTG, consider delivery if short-term variability is less than 3.5 or there are two successive non-reactive traces.
- Monitor with weekly multivessel Doppler, consider delivery if there are umbilical vein pulsations or reversed ductus venosus pulsations.
- Consider therapy with 40% humidified oxygen.

Key points for clinical practice

- The diagnosis of small for gestational age is usually based on an abdominal circumference or estimated fetal weight below the 10th centile.

Small for gestational age fetuses are at increased risk of perinatal mortality and morbidity, in addition to possible long-term health consequences.

Fetal abnormality should be excluded in some small for gestational age fetuses.

Umbilical artery Doppler is the single most important test for determining the at-risk small fetus. Randomised controlled trials have shown improved outcome without increasing intervention.

Monitoring growth velocity is important in the small fetus. Proper velocity measures should be used.

Further monitoring of the at-risk fetus may include assessment of liquor volume, cardiotocography, biophysical profile and multivessel Doppler waveform analysis.

The use of venous Doppler waveforms shows promise in assessment of the preterm fetus with abnormal umbilical artery Dopplers, but its value has yet to be evaluated in randomised controlled trials.

The timing of delivery remains controversial, but delivery before 32 weeks' gestation should only be considered where there is evidence of deterioration in fetal condition.

Maternal oxygen therapy shows promise as a treatment for early severe-growth restriction.

References

1. The GRIT Study Group. When do obstetricians recommend delivery for a high-risk preterm fetus? *Eur J Obstet Gynecol Reprod Biol* 1996; **67**: 121–126.
2. Cnattingius S, Haglund B, Kramer MS. Differences in late fetal death rates in association with different determinants of small for gestational age fetuses: population based cohort study. *BMJ* 1998; **316**: 1483–1487.
3. McIntyre DD, Bloom SL, Casey BM, Leveno KJ. Birth weight in relation to morbidity and mortality among newborn infants. *N Engl J Med* 1999; **340**: 1234–1238.
4. Strauss RS. Adult functional outcome of those born small for gestational age. Twenty–six-year follow-up of the 1970 British Birth Cohort. *JAMA* 2000; **283**: 625–632.
5. Morley R, Dwyer T. Fetal origins of adult disease? *Clin Exp Pharmacol Physiol* 2001; **28**: 962–966.
6. Neilson JP. Symphysis-fundal height measurement in pregnancy (Cochrane Review). Oxford: *The Cochrane Library*, Issue 2, 2002.
7. Chang TC, Robson SC, Boys RJ, Spencer JA. Prediction of the small for gestational age infant: which ultrasonic measurement is best? *Obstet Gynecol* 1992; **80**: 1030–1038.
8. Mongelli M, Gardosi J. Reduction of false-positive diagnosis of fetal growth restriction by application of customized fetal growth standards. *Obstet Gynecol* 1996; **88**: 844–848.
9. Chien PFW, Arnott N, Gordon A, Owen P, Khan KS. How useful is uterine artery Doppler flow velocimetry in the prediction of pre-eclampsia, intrauterine growth retardation and perinatal death? An overview. *Br J Obstet Gynaecol* 2000; **107**: 196–208.
10. Macara L, Kingdom JC, Kohnen G, Bowman AW, Greer IA, Kaufmann P. Elaboration of stem villous vessels in growth restricted pregnancies with abnormal umbilical artery Doppler waveforms. *Br J Obstet Gynaecol* 1995; **102**: 807–812.
11. Maulik D, Yarlagadda P, Youngblood JP, Ciston P. Comparative efficacy of umbilical arterial Doppler indices for predicting adverse perinatal outcome. *Am J Obstet Gynecol* 1991; **164**: 1434–1438.
12. Karsdorp VH, van Vugt JM, van Geijn HP *et al*. Clinical significance of absent or reversed end diastolic velocity waveforms in umbilical artery. *Lancet* 1994: **344**: 1664–1668.
13. Trudinger BJ, Cook CM, Giles WB *et al*. Fetal umbilical artery velocity waveforms and subsequent neonatal outcome. *Br J Obstet Gynaecol* 1991; **98**: 378–384.
14. Ozcan T, Sbracia R, d'Ancona RL, Copel JA, Mari G. Arterial and venous Doppler velocimetry in the severely growth-restricted fetus and associations with adverse perinatal outcome. *Ultrasound Obstet Gynecol* 1998; **39**: 39–44.
15. Baschat AA, Gembruch U, Harman CR. The sequence of changes in Doppler and biophysical parameters as severe fetal growth restriction worsens. *Ultrasound Obstet Gynecol* 2001; **18**: 571–577.
16. Hecher K, Bilardo CM, Stigter RH *et al*. Monitoring of fetuses with intrauterine growth restriction: a longitudinal study. *Ultrasound Obstet Gynecol* 2001; **18**: 564–570.
17. Sickler GK, Nyberg DA, Sohaey R, Luthy DA. Polyhydramnios and fetal intrauterine growth restriction: ominous combination. *J Ultrasound Med* 1997; **16**: 609–614.
18. Magann EF, Sanderson M, Martin JN, Chauhan S. The amniotic fluid index, single deepest pocket, and two-diameter pocket in normal human pregnancy. *Am J Obstet Gynecol* 2000; **182**: 1581–1588.
19. Owen P, Mires GJ, Christie AD. Impaired fetal growth velocity in the presence of notched uterine artery velocity waveforms. *Br J Obstet Gynaecol* 1996; **103**: 1247–1249.
20. Alfirevic Z, Neilson JP. Doppler ultrasonography in high-risk pregnancies: systematic review with meta-analysis. *Am J Obstet Gynecol* 1995; **172**: 1379–1387.
21. Neilson JP, Alfirevic Z. Doppler ultrasound for fetal assessment of high risk pregnancies (Cochrane Review). Oxford: *The Cochrane Library*, Issue 2, 2002.
22. Pattison N, McCowan L. Cardiotocography for antepartum fetal assessment (Cochrane Review). Oxford: *The Cochrane Library*, Issue 2, 2002.
23. Walkinshaw SA, McPhail S, Cameron H, Robson SC. The prediction of fetal compromise and acidosis by biophysical profile scoring in the small for gestational age fetus. *J Perinat Med* 1992; **20**: 345–350.
24. Mari G, Deter RL. Middle cerebral artery flow velocity waveforms in normal and small-for-gestational-age fetuses. *Am J Obstet Gynecol* 1992; **166**: 1262–1270.

25. Gugmundsson S, Tulzer G, Huhta JC, Marsal K. Venous Doppler in the fetus with absent end-diastolic flow in the umbilical artery. *Ultrasound Obstet Gynecol* 1996; **7**: 262–267.
26. Sicco A. Neurodevelopmental outcome at 3 years of age after fetal 'brain sparing'. *Early Hum Dev* 1998; **52**: 67–79.
27. Hecher K, Hackeloer BJ. Cardiotocogram compared to Doppler investigation of the fetal circulation in the premature growth-retarded fetus: longitudinal observations. *Ultrasound Obstet Gynecol* 1997; **9**: 152–161.
28. Baschat AA, Gembruch U, Reiss I, Gortner L, Weiner CP, Harman CR. Relationship between arterial and venous Doppler and perinatal outcome in fetal growth restriction. *Ultrasound Obstet Gynecol* 2000; **16**: 407–414.
29. Nicolaides KH, Campbell S, Bradley RJ, Bilardo CM, Soothill PW, Gibb D. Maternal oxygen therapy for intrauterine growth retardation. *Lancet* 1987; **1**: 942–945.
30. Lindow SW, Mantel GD, Anthony J, Coetzee EJ. A double-blind randomised controlled trial of continuous oxygen therapy for compromised fetuses. *Br J Obstet Gynaecol* 2002; **109**: 509–513.

Mark D. Kilby   Katherine J. Barber

5

Management of abnormal liver function in pregnancy

Liver dysfunction complicates as many as 3% of pregnancies.[1] Liver disease in pregnancy can effect both maternal and fetal health. Hypertensive disease of pregnancy, which encompasses the spectrum of pre-eclampsia and HELLP syndrome, accounted for 16 maternal deaths in the UK between 1997–1999. Two deaths were from hepatic rupture as a complication of severe pre-eclampsia – five deaths were associated with HELLP syndrome.[2] Likewise, acute fatty liver of pregnancy (AFLP) continues to cause small numbers of maternal deaths.[2] Intrahepatic cholestasis of pregnancy causes maternal morbidity and is responsible for significant fetal mortality and morbidity.[3]

PHYSIOLOGICAL CHANGES

Anatomically, the liver does not change in size during pregnancy but is more difficult to palpate due to rotation to a more superior and posterior position.[4] During pregnancy, blood flow through the liver remains unaltered.[5] The increased circulating volume in pregnancy is redistributed through the portal veins and vena cava resulting in the appearance of engorgement of the oesophageal veins at endoscopy in 50% of normal pregnancies.[6]

Pregnancy-induced physiological changes in liver metabolism are shown in Table 1. A study in 1997 of measured aspartate transaminase (AST), alanine aminotransferase (ALT), bilirubin and γ-glutamyltransferase (γ-GT) in 430 apparently normal pregnant women reported these indices to be approximately 20% lower in pregnant women compared to laboratory reference ranges.[7] Total serum protein concentration also decreases, mainly due to a 25%

Mark D. Kilby MD MRCOG, Professor of Maternal and Fetal Medicine, Department of Fetal Medicine, Division of Reproduction and Child Health, Birmingham Women's Hospital, University of Birmingham, Edgbaston, Birmingham B15 2TG, UK (for correspondence)

Katherine J. Barber MB ChB MRCOG, Wellcome Research Fellow, Department of Reproduction and Child Health, University of Birmingham, Edgbaston, Birmingham B15 2TG, UK

Table 1 Normal values and pregnancy specific reference ranges for liver function tests

Liver function test	Non-pregnant range	Pregnancy specific reference ranges, by trimester[17]		
		1st trimester	2nd trimester	3rd trimester
AST (IU/l)	7–40	10–28	11–29	11–30
ALT (IU/l)	0–40	6–32	6–32	6–32
APL (IU/l)	20–125	60–375		
Bilirubin	0–17	4–16	3–13	3–14
γ-GT (IU/l)	7–41	5–37	4–43	3–41
Albumin (g/l)	35–55	Falls by 10 g/l mostly in 1st trimester		
Total protein (g/l)	65–80	Falls by 10 g/l by 16–20th week		
Globulin (g/l)	30–50	Increases progressively to term		
Fibrinogen (g/l)	2–4	Increases progressively to term		

fall in serum albumin concentration, secondary to haemodilution occurring as a result of expansion of circulating volume. Alkaline phosphatase (ALP) increases 2–4-fold because of synthesis by the syncytiotophoblast. The concentrations of liver-derived clotting factors (fibrinogen, prothrombin and Factors VII, VIII, IX and X) are dramatically increased which decreases *in vitro* clotting studies, such as prothrombin and partial thromboplastin times.

Liver function continues to alter into the puerperium. Serum transaminases show a gradual increase in the first 2–5 post-natal days and mode of delivery, methods of analgesia, maternal age and breast feeding also influence liver function tests.

Liver disease in pregnancy can be considered in three categories: (i) disease peculiar to pregnancy; (ii) pre-existing and co-incidental disease; and (iii) hepatobilliary disease.

JAUNDICE/LIVER DYSFUNCTION CAUSED BY PREGNANCY

PRE-HEPATIC CAUSES

Haemolysis: pre-eclampsia and HELLP syndrome

Pre-eclampsia causes pre-hepatic dysfunction in association with HELLP syndrome (micro-angiopathic haemolysis, elevated liver transaminases and low platelets). HELLP complicates pre-eclampsia in 4–12% of cases.[8] The overall incidence of HELLP in a prospective study of 12,068 pregnant women was found to be 0.11%.[9]

Fetal disorders of mitochondrial fatty acid oxidation have recently been associated with obstetric complications including pre-eclampsia, HELLP syndrome, placental bed infarct, and acute fatty liver of pregnancy (AFLP). These disorders occur in about one-third of mothers who are heterozygous for a defect in the long-chain 3-hydroxyacyl-CoA dehydrogenase (LCHAD) enzyme and who bear a fetus homozygous for the defect.[10] The mechanism is not understood.

In the majority of women, HELLP syndrome arises in the third trimester usually in association with pre-eclampsia. Patients with hypertension may present principally with hepatic dysfunction. Symptoms such as nausea, epigastric or right upper quadrant pain, headache and visual disturbance are in common with those of pre-eclampsia. Clinical deterioration may be rapid leading to disseminated intravascular coagulation (DIC), renal failure, adult respiratory distress syndrome (ARDS) and hepatic haemorrhage. Following delivery, there may be serious initial deterioration, rather than improvement.

A report on 54 maternal deaths from HELLP syndrome in the US revealed that causes of death included cerebral haemorrhage (45%), cardiopulmonary arrest (40%), disseminated intravascular coagulopathy (39%), adult respiratory distress syndrome (28%), renal failure (28%), sepsis (23%), hepatic haemorrhage (20%), and hypoxic ischaemic encephalopathy (16%). Delay in diagnosis of HELLP syndrome was implicated in 22 of 43 patients' deaths (51.1%).[11] The recent *Confidential Enquiry into Maternal Mortality* in the UK reported deaths from HELLP syndrome where deterioration was rapid from fulminant disease.[2]

Patients with pre-eclampsia should routinely be screened for HELLP syndrome with tests of liver function and platelet count. Elevated serum transaminases are part of HELLP syndrome.[12] With significant liver involvement, coagulation abnormalities develop. Fetal well-being and growth should be assessed since placental insufficiency occurs in about 30% of pre-eclamptic patients.[13] Intra-uterine growth restriction is usually asymmetrical, with brain development spared at the expense of abdominal girth.

The patient with hepatic involvement should be managed at a centre with intensive care facilities, with blood products (including coagulation factors, cryoprecipitate and platelets) readily available, and laboratory facilities geared to rapid analysis and reporting of results.[2] The multidisciplinary team should consist of a consultant obstetrician, anaesthetist, haematologist, hepatologist and neonatologist.[2]

When liver involvement is suspected, ultrasonography may delineate an intrahepatic haematoma.[14] Liver and renal function should be measured serially. Eclampsia complicating HELLP and severe pre-eclampsia should be anticipated and prophylactic magnesium sulphate treatment should be considered.[15]

Antenatal steroid therapy with intramuscular betamethasone or dexamethasone is advised prior to delivery of a preterm fetus. The administration of glucocorticoids to patients with HELLP syndrome, both antenatally and postnatally, can shorten disease course, reduce recovery times, and decrease morbidity. A randomised controlled trial in 40 antenatal patients with HELLP syndrome showed that intravenous dexamethasone (10 mg given 12-hourly) was more effective than intramuscular betamethasone (12 mg given 24-hourly) in improving liver dysfunction and thrombocytopenia, and stabilising hypertension.[16]

Disseminated intravascular coagulation (DIC)
Activation of the coagulation system may arise from the events listed in Table 2. Intravascular coagulation results in the deposition of fibrin, which may obstruct small vessels leading to organ dysfunction, including hepatic dysfunction.

The removal of the triggering factor for DIC (*e.g.* delivery in placental abruption) coupled with supportive treatment in the form of replacement of blood components, monitoring of coagulation times, renal and liver function,

Table 2 Mechanisms triggering DIC in pregnancy

Trigger of DIC	Disease of pregnancy
Endothelial injury	Pre-eclampsia, septicaemia, hypovolaemia
Thromboplastin	Placental abruption, amniotic fluid embolism, intra-uterine death (retained fetus), intra-uterine sepsis, hydatidiform mole
Phospholipid	Intravascular haemolysis, large feto–maternal haemorrhage, septicaemia

circulatory support, and adequate oxygenation requires multidisciplinary co-operation between obstetricians, haematologists and anaesthetists.

Sepsis

Abnormal liver function may arise with Gram-negative septicaemia (*e.g. Escherichia coli*), urinary tract infection,[1] and chorio-amnionitis. Treatment of the underlying infection results in the rapid return of normal liver function.

Subcapsular haemorrhage

Subcapsular haemorrhage is associated with severe pre-eclampsia and HELLP syndrome and carries a poor prognosis. Deposits of fibrin-like material occur in the hepatic sinusoids which impair hepatic blood flow leading to swelling of the liver and coagulopathy associated with HELLP. A more detailed explanation follows.

HEPATIC CAUSES PECULIAR TO PREGNANCY

Hepatic ischaemia, necrosis and hepatic rupture

In pre-eclampsia and HELLP syndrome, classic lesions in the liver are periportal or focal parenchymal necrosis and periportal 'lake' haemorrhages.[18] Deposits of fibrin-like material may obstruct blood flow in sinusoids in severe pre-eclampsia leading to swelling of the liver and hepatic capsular distension. This causes epigastric pain. Haemorrhage can occur beneath the capsule and, rarely, rupture of the capsule may occur with fatal consequences. Infarction and rupture can occur at any time including the puerperium, causing severe epigastric pain, profound hypovolaemic shock, fetal demise, haemorrhagic diathesis and hepatic encephalopathy. As hepatocellular damage occurs, intracellular hepatic enzymes (*e.g.* AST, ALT) are released into the circulation and hepatic synthesis is impaired, reflected in the increased prothrombin time.

Rapid resuscitation is required with intravenous fluids, blood transfusion and coagulation factors as well as surgical repair of the liver (oversewing, packing, hepatic artery ligation or partial hepatectomy). If rupture occurs antenatally, fetal survival is unlikely.

Acute fatty liver of pregnancy (AFLP)

AFLP is a rare, but potentially fatal, complication in the third trimester of pregnancy. The morbidity and mortality of this disorder has decreased significantly in recent

Table 3 Abnormal investigations in AFLP

Elevated bilirubin
Elevated transaminases
Hypoglycaemia
Elevated urate
Elevated ammonia
Renal impairment
Leukocytosis
Coagulopathy
Ascites or bright liver on ultrasound
Microvesicular steatosis on liver biopsy

years with recognition and aggressive management. Recommended treatment is expeditious delivery with maximal supportive care.

The multisystem liver involvement in pre-eclampsia may overlap with acute fatty liver of pregnancy. Both conditions tend to improve with delivery and share clinical manifestations and laboratory abnormalities.[4] AFLP is characterised histologically by the accumulation of microvesicular fat within hepatocytes (microvesicular steatosis). Macrovesicles of fat are more common in other liver diseases.[19]

The reported incidence of AFLP from retrospective analyses is between 1 in 9000 and 1 in 13,000. A recent series reported a low maternal and fetal mortality.[20]

AFLP usually presents in the third trimester with nausea, vomiting, anorexia and malaise of gradual onset. Mild features of pre-eclampsia may co-exist. There may be polydipsia and polyuria in the absence of diabetes, abdominal pain and encephalopathy. Jaundice may occur 2 or 3 weeks following the onset of these symptoms. Abnormal investigations due to AFLP are listed in Table 3. The incidence of AFLP has been found to be increased in women who carry a fetus with a defect in fatty acid oxidation, and who are themselves carriers of a genetic mutation which reduces the activity of the trifunctional protein (TP) of fatty acid oxidation[21] that partially compromises their own intramitochondrial fatty acid oxidation pathway.[22]

The management of acute fatty liver of pregnancy involves maternal stabilisation followed by delivery and supportive care. Early recognition and intervention can result in excellent maternal and fetal outcomes. Fetal assessment with heart rate monitoring and ultrasound assessment of biophysical profile are recommended because of the increased risk of fetal distress or still-birth in pregnancies complicated by acute fatty liver of pregnancy. The principles of management are common to those of HELLP syndrome.

Hyperemesis gravidarum

Liver dysfunction in hyperemesis gravidarum arises in up to 25% of affected pregnancies.[23] AST may be elevated but liver synthesis remains intact. Normal liver function quickly returns once adequate rehydration and nutrition has been instituted.[24] Intramuscular corticosteroids have also been used to treat severe hyperemesis although a small randomised-controlled study failed to show any statistically significant benefit.[25]

POST-HEPATIC CAUSES OF HEPATIC DYSFUNCTION PECULIAR TO PREGNANCY

Obstetric cholestasis

Obstetric cholestasis (OC), also known as intrahepatic cholestasis of pregnancy, is one of the primary disorders of the liver that adversely affects maternal well-being and fetal outcome. Early identification of this condition, careful interdisciplinary monitoring, and prompt delivery at fetal maturity can improve outcomes in the mother and child. OC also predisposes to gallstones. The incidence of OC varies from 0.1% to 1.5% of pregnancies in Europe. A recent prospective study in the UK found the incidence to be 0.6%.[1]

OC probably arises from a genetic predisposition for increased sensitivity to oestrogens and progestogens, and altered membrane composition and expression of bile ducts, hepatocytes, and canalicular transport systems.[26] The elevation in maternal levels of bile acids impairs the normal feto–maternal transfer and excess bile acids with abnormal profiles accumulate which are toxic to the fetus.[27]

OC presents usually in the second half of pregnancy. Pruritus is the chief complaint and generally starts in the palms and soles, progresses to the arms and legs, and eventually involves the trunk and face. The pruritus leads to sleep deprivation. Jaundice may occur and typically develops 1–4 weeks after the onset of pruritus. Subclinical steatorrhoea may also be present along with vitamin K deficiency due to fat malabsorption, leading to postpartum haemorrhage. In 40–60% of subsequent pregnancies, the condition recurs in affected women.[28] OC is associated with preterm delivery, increased perinatal mortality, intrapartum non-reassuring fetal heart rate patterns, and meconium staining of the amniotic fluid. In pregnancies complicated with OC, premature births occur in up to 60%, fetal distress in up to 33% and intra-uterine death in up to 2% of cases.[3] When untreated, perinatal mortality ranges from 11–20%.[29] Cardiotocographs (CTGs) have been reported as being normal up to 2 days before fetal demise.[29]

Liver function tests show elevated serum bile acids and γ-GT levels may be increased. A recent Cochrane review evaluating the effectiveness and safety of ursodeoxycholic acid, guar gum, S-adenosylmethionine and activated charcoal found insufficient evidence to recommend any of these therapies for treatment of OC. Most fetal deaths occur late in pregnancy, after 36 weeks of gestation, hence the rationale for effecting delivery early if fetal lung maturity is attained.

Acute pancreatitis of pregnancy

Peak incidence of pancreatitis is in the third trimester coinciding with peak levels of circulating type 5 triglycerides.[30] Cholelithiasis, which sometimes causes pancreatitis, is more common in pregnancy. Methyldopa, commonly prescribed in pregnancy, may cause pancreatitis.

Constant, severe epigastric pain radiating through to the back is the classical presentation of acute pancreatitis. Serum amylase levels are typically 5 times greater than the normal, and abnormal liver function reflects the severity of the disease. Mortality in pregnancy is uncommon and fetal demise is around 10% is reported.

All but the most severe cases respond to conservative management with strict fluid balance using colloid and crystalloid infusion, correction of electrolyte imbalance, and restriction of oral intake. Surgical intervention is not usually required, but pancreatic debridement may be necessary in cases refractory to medical management.

LIVER DISEASE COINCIDENTAL TO PREGNANCY

HAEMOLYSIS

Sickle cell disease
Liver and biliary tract dysfunction are common complications of sickle cell anaemia. The disorders are related to haemolysis, anaemia and transfusion management, and the consequences of sickling and vaso-occlusion.

Chronic haemolysis and accelerated bilirubin turnover leads to a high incidence of pigment gallstones and biliary sludge. In addition to biliary colic, this predisposes to cholecystitis and pancreatitis. Complications of repeated blood transfusion include transmission of hepatitis B and C. Measurement of antibodies to these viruses should be performed antenatally.

Prophylactic transfusion for anaemia exacerbated by pregnancy is controversial, unless other complications co-exist, such as severe anaemia, pre-eclampsia, or increased frequency of painful crises. Iron overload occurs with frequent transfusion which can lead to haemochromatosis.

Painful vaso-occlusive crises affect the liver causing right upper quadrant pain, fever, jaundice, elevated AST/ALT and hepatic enlargement. Treatment is supportive.

Malaria
Haemolysis due to the malaria parasite frequently causes jaundice. Pregnant women are especially at-risk from malaria because the malarial parasite favours the placenta as a site of parasite accumulation. At least 24 million pregnancies are affected by malaria annually in Africa and malaria causes up to 15% of maternal anaemia and about 35% of preventable low birth-weight. The management of uncomplicated falciparum malaria comprises specific antimalarial drugs and supportive therapy. Hepatic failure is rare.

Iatrogenic (heart valves)
Mechanical trauma to red blood cells by prosthetic heart valves may cause haemolytic disease with anaemia, jaundice, and congestive cardiac failure. Treatment involves assessing valvular and cardiac function, as well as iron therapy to correct anaemia

INHERITED DISORDERS OF BILIRUBIN METABOLISM

Gilbert's syndrome, Dubin-Johnson syndrome, and Rotor syndrome
This group of hyperbilirubinaemias are relatively benign causing life-long mild, asymptomatic jaundice. They are caused by deficiencies in bilirubin conjugation (Gilbert's syndrome) and bile transporters (Dubin-Johnson and Rotor syndromes). Jaundice may be exacerbated in pregnancy and by the combined oral contraceptive pill. Treatment is usually unnecessary and fetal outcomes are good.

Table 4 Serological antibodies and markers of acute viral hepatitis

Virus	Antibodies	Other markers
Hepatitis A	IgM antihepatitis A virus	
Hepatitis B	IgM antihepatitis B core antigen (HBc)	Hepatitis B virus DNA clearance
	Presence of hepatitis Be anti-gen (Hbe) indicates replication and active infection	
Hepatitis C	IgM antihepatitis C virus	Hepatitis C RNA detection by PCR
Hepatitis D	IgM antihepatitis D	Hepatitis D virus RNA clearance
Hepatitis E	IgM antihepatitis E	Hepatitis E virus RNA clearance
Herpes viruses (simplex, zoster, cytomegalovirus, Epstein-Barr)	IgM antibodies	Cultures, paired sera, and *in situ* hybridisation

DRUG-RELATED HEPATIC DYSFUNCTION

Paracetamol
Paracetamol overdose is often fatal, secondary to fulminant hepatic failure, and is the commonest cause of acute liver failure in the UK. The toxic metabolite causes irreversible hepatotoxicity. Treatment with N-acetylcysteine is advised.

Alcohol
Alcohol-induced hepatic dysfunction is uncommon in pregnancy.

BUDD-CHIARI SYNDROME (THROMBOPHILIAS)

In this rare syndrome, the venous outflow of the liver is obstructed with occlusion of the hepatic vein. Thrombophilias such as activated protein C deficiency due to Factor V Leiden mutation predispose to this condition in pregnancy. Acute hepatic venous occlusion presents with abdominal pain, vomiting, tender hepatomegally and ascites. Liver transplantation is the treatment of choice.

VIRAL HEPATITIS

Viral hepatitis is the commonest cause of jaundice in pregnancy.[4] The principal viruses infecting the liver are shown in Table 4.

Hepatitis A
Hepatitis A virus is a RNA virus spread predominantly by the faecal-oral route. Exposure is usually in childhood and the disease is usually mild, consisting of influenza-like symptoms. Cholestatic jaundice with pruritis, dark

urine and pale stools develops within a few days. Liver function tests reveal normal alkaline phosphatase and γ-GT, with elevated aspartate transaminase and alanine transaminase. Differentiation from other causes of jaundice presenting in pregnancy may be difficult and testing for hepatitis A IgM is required to exclude it. Management is supportive only and the disease is not more severe in pregnancy.

Hepatitis B

Hepatitis B (HBV) affects more than 350 million people world-wide and is transmitted in blood and serum mainly by sexual intercourse, blood transfusion and intravenous drug use. Acute infection can be relatively asymptomatic and without jaundice. However, 1–10% of healthy adults and over 90% of infected babies may fail to clear the virus and become chronic carriers of the virus.[4] Cirrhosis, liver failure, or hepatocellular carcinoma will develop in approximately 15–40% of infected patients. In the West, the incidence of chronic carrier status is 0.5–5% of the population.[23]

The relevance to maternal–fetal medicine is the high risk of vertical transmission, the predisposition of the infected neonate to become a chronic carrier, and the potential for eradication by immunisation. In the UK, it is recommended that the antenatal population should be screened for HBV so that immunisation can be instituted for the offspring of carriers.[31,32] National guidelines advise that: (i) all women have information on, and access to, HBV screening as part of their antenatal care; and (ii) all babies born to mothers with HBV infection receive immunisation at or as soon after birth.

There is no contra-indication to vaginal delivery. Breast-feeding of infants of chronic HBV carriers causes no additional risk for the transmission of the hepatitis B virus.

Hepatitis C

Infection with hepatitis C (HCV) occurs world-wide, with a prevalence of antibody to HCV (anti-HCV) in serum in most industrialised countries of 1–2%. Hepatitis C is a blood-borne viral infection that was discovered in the context of blood transfusion. Most Western countries screen donated blood for hepatitis C. Injection-drug abuse accounts for most new infections in the US. HCV may also be transmitted from about 5% of infected mothers to their infant.

Most patients with acute infection are symptom-free and only a small proportion become jaundiced. HCV infection becomes chronic in about 85% of individuals as demonstrated by the persistence of HCV RNA in serum. Virtually all patients with chronic HCV infection develop histological features of chronic hepatitis and around 20% of patients develop cirrhosis in the first or second decade of HCV infection. Unlike with hepatitis B there is no means of immunising a neonate against the vertical transmission of hepatitis C.

Hepatitis D

Hepatitis D is an incomplete RNA virus that requires hepatitis B surface antigen to transmit its genome from cell to cell. It only occurs in patients that are positive for hepatitis B surface antigen and is mainly confined to intravenous drug users in the UK.

Hepatitis E

Hepatitis E causes epidemic, enteric infection in the non-industrialised world and is extremely rare in the UK. The illness is similar to hepatitis A, but, in 15% of pregnant women, fulminant liver failure is reported.

AUTOIMMUNE DISEASE: CHRONIC ACTIVE HEPATITIS

Chronic active hepatitis in women of reproductive age may have autoimmune features with smooth muscle antibodies, nuclear factor (ANF) and auto-antibodies to specific proteins. Some are due to Wilson's disease, viral hepatitis, and drugs including methyldopa. Untreated chronic active hepatitis is associated with amenorrhoea and infertility. Flare-up of chronic active hepatitis has been reported during pregnancy. Drugs used to treat chronic active hepatitis (e.g. prednisolone and azathioprine) may be used during pregnancy without ill effect on the fetus. Pregnant women with chronic active hepatitis have a higher incidence of still-births and low birth-weight infants.

INHERITED LIVER DISEASES

Primary biliary cirrhosis

Primary biliary cirrhosis (PBC) is an organ-specific autoimmune disease that predominantly affects women and is characterised by chronic progressive destruction of small intrahepatic bile ducts with portal inflammation and ultimately fibrosis. The serological hallmark of PBC is the presence of antibodies to mitochondria. Treatment is symptomatic and vitamin K supplements should be given.

Wilson's disease (hepatolenticular degeneration)

Wilson's disease is rare, autosomal recessive condition characterised by the deposition of copper in the brain, liver, cornea and other organs. Clinical features include liver cirrhosis, liver failure, neurological dysfunction and intellectual deterioration. Pregnant patients with Wilson's disease should remain on anti-copper therapy with zinc during pregnancy.

Haemochromatosis

Haemochromatosis is an autosomal recessive condition, affecting around 1 in 300 Caucasians. Iron is absorbed in excess and deposited in various organs including the liver leading to eventual fibrosis and functional organ failure. Cirrhosis is a late feature in untreated individuals. Venesection relieves iron overload, prolongs life and may reverse tissue damage.

CIRRHOSIS

Pregnancy in advanced cirrhosis is rare and fetal loss is high.[4] Maternal prognosis depends on the degree of hepatic dysfunction. Bleeding from oesophageal varices is the most significant complication, and most likely in the first trimester. Vitamin supplementation is essential.

POST-HEPATIC CAUSES OF LIVER DYSFUNCTION

Cholelithiasis

Gallstones and pancreatitis are two non-obstetric causes of abdominal pain and abnormal liver function tests. Typically, liver function tests will show an obstructive picture. Gallbladder surgery in pregnancy is second only to that for acute appendicitis. Endoscopic cholecystectomy can successfully be performed in the first and second trimesters, but is technically more difficult in late pregnancy.

Cholangiocarcinoma

Cholangiocarcinomas can be either intra- or extrahepatic: extrahepatic tumours give rise to post-hepatic jaundice. The prognosis for these tumours is poor.

Cholangitis

Acute cholangitis is due to bacterial infection in the biliary tree and is always secondary to bile duct abnormalities (*e.g.* bile duct stones, biliary strictures, neoplasms). The symptoms are fever, upper abdominal pain and jaundice. Gram-negative septicaemia may develop. Treatment is with intravenous antibiotics and fluids.

Inflammatory bowel disease

Crohn's disease and ulcerative colitis affect 3–7 per 100,000 and 6–10 per 100,000 of the population in Western countries, respectively. A considerable proportion of patients with inflammatory bowel disease have abnormal liver function tests. Pregnancy neither relieves nor exacerbates inflammatory bowel disease.

Key points for clinical practice

- Liver dysfunction arises in up to 3% of pregnancies.

- Patients with pre-eclampsia should be screened for HELLP syndrome with liver function tests and platelet count.

- For patients with hepatic involvement, a multidisciplinary team is required, with intensive care facilities and ready availability of blood products.

- Acute fatty liver of pregnancy presents in the third trimester with malaise of gradual onset followed by jaundice. Early recognition and delivery with supportive care usually results in good maternal and fetal outcome.

- Obstetric cholestasis presents in the second half of pregnancy with progressive pruritus which may be followed by jaundice. Most fetal deaths occur after 36 weeks of gestation; therefore, early delivery when fetal lungs are mature should be considered.

- Viral hepatitis is the commonest cause of jaundice in pregnancy. Antenatal screening for hepatitis B (HBV) is recommended to enable immunisation of all babies born to mothers with HBV.

References

1. Ch'ng CL, Morgan M, Hainsworth I, Kingham J. Prospective study of liver dysfunction in pregnancy in Southwest Wales. *Gut* 2002; **51**: 876–880.
2. Department of Health. *Why Mothers Die. Report on Confidential Enquiries into Maternal Deaths in the United Kingdom 1997–99.* London: Stationary Office; 2002.
3. Lammert F, Marschall H, Glantz A, Matern S. Intrahepatic cholestasis of pregnancy: molecular pathogenesis, diagnosis and management. *J Hepatol* 2000; **33**:1012–1021.
4. Fagan EA. Diseases of the liver, biliary system and pancreas. In: Creasy RK, Resnik RP. (eds) *Maternal–Fetal Medicine. Principles and Practice.* Philadelphia, PA: WB Saunders, 1986; 1040–1061.
5. Chesley LC. Cardiovascular changes in pregnancy. *Obstet Gynecol Annu* 1975; **4**: 71–97.
6. Britton RC. Pregnancy and esophageal varices. *Am J Surg* 1982; **143**: 421–425.
7. van Thiel D. Effects of pregnancy and sex hormones on the liver. *Semin Liver Dis* 1987; **7**: 1–66.
8. Rahman TM, Wendon J. Severe hepatic dysfunction in pregnancy. *Q J Med* 2002; **95**: 343–357.
9. Abraham KA, Connolly G, Farrell J, Walshe JJ. The HELLP syndrome, a prospective study. *Ren Fail* 2001; **23**: 705–713.
10. Tyni T, Ekholm E, Pihko H. Pregnancy complications are frequent in long-chain 3-hydroxyacyl-coenzyme A dehydrogenase deficiency. *Am J Obstet Gynecol* 1998; **178**: 603–608.
11. Isler CM, Rinehart BK, Terrone DA, Martin RW, Magann EF, Martin Jr JN. Maternal mortality associated with HELLP (hemolysis, elevated liver enzymes, and low platelets) syndrome. *Am J Obstet Gynecol* 1999; **181**: 924–928.
12. Saphier CJ, Repke JT. Hemolysis, elevated liver enzymes, and low platelets (HELLP) syndrome: a review of diagnosis and management. *Semin Perinatol* 1998; **22**: 118–133.
13. Walker JJ. Pre-eclampsia. *Lancet* 2000; **356**: 1260–1265.
14. Chan AD, Gerscovich EO. Imaging of subcapsular hepatic and renal hematomas in pregnancy complicated by pre-eclampsia and the HELLP syndrome. *J Clin Ultrasound* 1999; **27**: 35–40.
15. Anon. Do women with pre-eclampsia, and their babies, benefit from magnesium sulphate? The Magpie Trial: a randomised placebo-controlled trial. *Lancet* 2002; **359**: 1877–1890.
16. Isler CM, Barrilleaux PS, Magann EF, Bass JD, Martin Jr JN. A prospective, randomized trial comparing the efficacy of dexamethasone and betamethasone for the treatment of antepartum HELLP (hemolysis, elevated liver enzymes, and low platelet count) syndrome. *Am J Obstet Gynecol* 2001; **184**: 1332–1337.
17. Girling JC, Dow E, Smith JH. Liver function tests in pre-eclampsia: importance of comparison with a reference range derived for normal pregnancy. *Br J Obstet Gynaecol* 1997; **104**: 246–250.
18. Walker JJ. Current thoughts on the pathophysiology of pre-eclampsia/eclampsia. In: Studd J. (ed) *Progress in Obstetrics and Gynaecology*, vol. 13. Edinburgh: Churchill Livingstone, 1998; 177–190.
19. Ockner SA, Brunt EM, Cohn SM, Krul ES, Hanto DW, Peters MG. Fulminant hepatic failure caused by acute fatty liver of pregnancy treated by orthoptic liver transplantation. *Hepatology* 1990; **11**: 59–64.
20. Castro MA, Fassett MJ, Reynolds TB, Shaw KJ, Goodwin TM. Reversible peripartum liver failure: a new perspective on the diagnosis, treatment, and cause of acute fatty liver of pregnancy, based on 28 consecutive cases. *Am J Obstet Gynecol* 1999; **181**: 389–395.
21. Strauss AW, Bennett MJ, Rinaldo P *et al.* Inherited long-chain 3-hydroxyacyl-CoA dehydrogenase deficiency and a fetal-maternal interaction cause maternal liver disease and other pregnancy complications. *Semin Perinatol* 1999; **23**: 100–112.
22. Ibdah JA, Bennett MJ, Rinaldo P *et al.* A fetal fatty-acid oxidation disorder as a cause of liver disease in pregnant women. *N Engl J Med* 1999; **340**: 1723–1731.
23. Fagan EA. Disorders of liver, biliary system and pancreas. In: de Swiet M. (ed) *Medical Disorders in Obstetric Practice.* London: Blackwell Science, 1995; 321–379.
24. Larrey D, Rueff B, Feldmann G, Degott C, Danan G, Benhamou JP. Recurrent jaundice caused by recurrent hyperemesis gravidarum. *Gut* 1984; **25**: 1414–1415.

25. Nelson-Piercy C, Fayers P, de Swiet M. Randomised, double-blind, placebo-controlled trial of corticosteroids for the treatment of hyperemesis gravidarum. *Br J Obstet Gynaecol* 2001; **108**: 9–15.

26. Milkiewicz P, Elias E, Williamson C, Weaver J. Obstetric cholestasis. *BMJ* 2002; **324**: 123–124.

27. Mazzella G, Rizzo N, Azzaroli F *et al*. Ursodeoxycholic acid administration in patients with cholestasis of pregnancy: effects on primary bile acids in babies and mothers. *Hepatology* 2001; **33**: 504–508.

28. Reyes H, Sjovall J. Bile acids and progesterone metabolites in intrahepatic cholestasis of pregnancy. *Ann Med* 2000; **32**: 94–106.

29. Rioseco AJ, Ivankovic MB, Manzur A *et al*. Intrahepatic cholestasis of pregnancy: a retrospective case-control study of perinatal outcome. *Am J Obstet Gynecol* 1994; **170**: 890–895.

30. Loo CC, Tan JY. Decreasing the plasma triglyceride level in hypertriglyceridemia-induced pancreatitis in pregnancy: a case report. *Am J Obstet Gynecol* 2002; **187**: 241–242.

31. NHS Executive. *Screening of Pregnant Women for Hepatitis B and Immunisation of Babies At Risk*. London: Department of Health (HSC 1998/127), 1998.

32. Department of Health and Royal College of Midwives. *Hepatitis B – Testing in Pregnancy*. London: Department of Health/Royal College of Midwives, 2000.

Michael S. Robson

6

Can the high Caesarean section rates be reduced?

Caesarean section rates have risen in many countries.[1,2] There is concern that the result will be a rise in complications without benefit to either mother or baby.[3] Three main issues need to be addressed in answering the question posed in the title: (i) justification for reducing a Caesarean section rate; (ii) acceptability to women of reducing a Caesarean section rate; and (iii) safe implementation of reducing a Caesarean section rate.

JUSTIFICATION

Any reduction of Caesarean section rates needs to be justified by the collection of accurate and up-to-date information, on a consistent and continuous basis, that monitors outcomes after all types of childbirth. This information should be available at both national and local levels and should be available for all outcomes before any attempt to reduce a Caesarean section rate is instigated. Caesarean section rates can be reduced, but can a Caesarean section rate be safely reduced? What evidence is required, and would that evidence be valid elsewhere? To justify reducing a Caesarean section rate, what constitutes a high Caesarean section rate needs to be defined. This can only be done by analysing the Caesarean section rate in detail in relation to other childbirth outcomes and available resources. Attempts should not be made to reduce a Caesarean section rate unless the other outcome factors are also kept under close scrutiny. To have a low Caesarean section rate as an ideal is as misguided as to have a high Caesarean section rate unless supported by data. Just as important as knowing how we might be able to reduce a high Caesarean section rate is knowing when and why a Caesarean section rate needs to be reduced and what the implications may be.

Michael S. Robson MBBS MRCOG FRCS Eng, Consultant Obstetrician and Gynaecologist, Wycombe General Hospital, High Wycombe, Buckinghamshire HP11 2TT, UK

INFORMATION

There are five main areas of outcome after childbirth where detailed information is required before we can interpret whether a Caesarean section rate is appropriate; (i) Caesarean section rates; (ii) maternal and perinatal morbidity and mortality rates; (iii) maternal satisfaction; (iv) medicolegal cases and complaints; and (v) available resources and expertise.

It is unclear where the responsibility for information collection lies, and the impact the Electronic Patient Record may have on the future collection and availability of that information. Successful, good quality, routine, information collection depends on the information being relevant, carefully defined, accurately collected, timely and available. The information collected needs to be organised or classified in a logical manner to transform crude data and information into useful knowledge that can improve clinical care.[4]

The purpose of a classification system determines the structure of the classification. The main groups of the classification should be robust enough that changes will be unlikely. The groups or categories of the classification should be **prospectively** identifiable so that outcome can be improved in those same patients in the future. The groups or categories must be mutually exclusive, totally inclusive and clinically relevant. The classification system must be simple to understand and easy to implement.[4]. These principles need to be applied in recording all of the childbirth outcomes in order to decide the appropriateness of a Caesarean section rate.

CAESAREAN SECTION RATES

For the last 30 years, there has been a public health concern about increasing Caesarean section rates. The increase has been a global phenomenon, the timing and rate of increase has differed from one country to another and marked differences in rates persist.[2] In 1985, the World Health Organization issued a consensus statement suggesting there were no additional health benefits associated with a Caesarean section rate above 10–15%. This was based on an examination of estimates of national Caesarean section rates and maternal and perinatal mortality rates from various countries. The advantages of a safe vaginal delivery over a Caesarean section are clear: safe vaginal delivery is associated with lower maternal and neonatal morbidity and costs less.

Caesarean section is considered by many as the most significant intervention in childbirth. The cost of a Caesarean section is significant. The cost of not doing one may also be significant. The justification of a Caesarean section is difficult to prove, not only in economic terms, but also in terms of maternal satisfaction and fetal and maternal morbidity and mortality. By any of these criteria, more detailed information about Caesarean sections is necessary and should be collected and returned centrally on a statutory, regular basis rather than by sporadic, small audits[2] using different definitions of childbirth outcomes.

Disagreement prevails amongst both women and professionals on Caesarean section rates. This disagreement suggests either inadequate information to answer the question, or the wrong questions being asked. Caesarean section rates will sometimes be too high and sometimes possibly too low. The Caesarean section rate will always be determined by fetal and maternal well-being, but ultimately will be a local decision, and appropriate Caesarean section rates may vary between different units. A Caesarean section rate can only be considered appropriate if the information is available to explain and justify it. Common to all professionals has been the problem of lack of information.

The number of Caesarean sections performed should be simple to determine, but the indications will be more difficult to standardise. Nevertheless, an attempt must be made. There should be one main indication, rather than a list of indications, using an agreed, standard hierarchical system. An example of this concept has been described.[5] Obstetricians then need to apply the methodology consistently. Indications for induction of labour should also be defined and standardised, as they often lead to Caesarean sections. A further point about data collection on Caesarean sections is that not only is the number of Caesarean sections performed important, but also, crucially, whether they have been performed on the right women at the right time and in an acceptable manner.

Accurate collection of data on Caesarean sections and the indications has to be continually emphasised. A balance between quantity and quality of data collection is required. An accurate, standardised, minimum data set is more important than large amounts of data, poorly collected. Information on Caesarean sections needs to be accurate, complete, up-to-date and available; not, as at present, often inaccurate, partially available, in an incomplete form many years later. Much of the work required at the present time involves defining the minimum data set expected and ensuring accurate, routine collection. The aim should not be to worry whether the Caesarean section rate is too high or too low, but rather what is the rate, why, and whether it can be considered to be appropriate, taking into consideration all the relevant outcome factors.[6] This assessment should be taking place on a continuous basis in all delivery units using whatever system they feel appropriate.

Caesarean sections do involve certain risks, but the operation is much safer than in previous years. At the same time, the increased awareness of the complications of vaginal delivery[7-10] and the increase in women's dissatisfaction with long labours and vaginal delivery have resulted in obstetricians having a lower threshold for advising delivery by Caesarean section.[11-13]

The Caesarean section rate is an important target, within the framework described, but should never be the only target and therefore never considered in isolation.

CLASSIFICATION OF CAESAREAN SECTIONS

There is no accepted classification system for Caesarean sections. An acceptable, simple system is required so that a Caesarean section rate can be analysed in more detail and explanations can be given for the Caesarean section rate and why it may have changed. Despite many descriptive studies, no standard classification system has been accepted that fits the principles of classification systems[4] and has been used prospectively to make changes in the management of labour in specific groups of women.[14] Caesarean section rates have been analysed by comparing overall rates, by indication for Caesarean

Table 1 The 10 group classification, Wycombe General Hospital 2001

Groups	Overall Caesarean section (CS) rate (%) – 545/2594 (21%)			
	No. CS over total No. women in each group	Relative size of groups (%)	CS rate in each group (%)	Contribution made by each group to the overall CS rate of 21%
1. Nulliparous, single cephalic, ≥ 37 weeks, in spontaneous labour	70/679	26.0 (679/2594)	10.3 (70/679)	2.7 (70/2594)
2. Nulliparous, single cephalic, ≥ 37 weeks, induced or CS before labour	105/281	10.8 (281/2594)	37.4 (105/281)	4.1 (105/2594)
3. Multiparous (excluding previous CS), single cephalic, ≥ 37 weeks, in spontaneous labour	21/866	33.4 (866/2594)	2.4 (21/866)	0.8 (21/2594)
4. Multiparous (excluding previous CS), single cephalic, ≥ 37 weeks, induced or CS before labour	33/224	8.6 (224/2594)	14.7 (33/224)	1.3 (33/2594)
5. Previous CS, single cephalic, → 37 weeks	141/214	8.2 (214/2594)	65.9 (141/214)	5.4 (141/2594)
6. All nulliparous breeches	43/47	1.8 (47/2594)	91.5 (43/47)	1.7 (43/2594)
7. All multiparous breeches (including previous CS)	49/59	2.3 (59/2594)	83.1 (49/59)	1.9 (49/2594)
8. All multiple pregnancies (including previous CS)	26/39	1.5 (39/2594)	66.7 (26/39)	1.0 (26/2594)
9. All abnormal lies (including previous CS)	8/8	0.3 (8/2594)	100 (8/8)	0.3 (8/2594)
10. All single cephalic, ≤ 36 weeks (including previous CS)	49/177	6.8 (177/2594)	27.7 (49/177)	1.9 (49/2594)

section,[15] by sub-groups of women,[16] and by primary and repeat Caesarean section rates; all have their disadvantages.[4]

The 10 group classification

The 10-group classification[4] has made possible comparisons of Caesarean section rates over time in one unit and between different units (Table 1). If implemented on a **continuous** basis, this classification would enable Caesarean section rates to be analysed with other childbirth outcomes and contribute to the assessment and justification of Caesarean section rates. The obstetric concepts, with their parameters, used to group and categorise the women in the 10-group classification are: the category of the pregnancy; the previous obstetric record of the woman; the course of labour and delivery; and the gestational age of the pregnancy. From these concepts and their parameters, the 10 groups were formed.

The concepts and their parameters are all prospective, mutually exclusive, totally inclusive, simple and easy to understand and organise (Table 2). They are clinically relevant to midwives and obstetricians because the information they depend on is required whenever an assessment is made of a pregnant woman who is either in labour or about to deliver. A pregnancy can only be single cephalic, single breech, multiple or a transverse or oblique lie (category of pregnancy). A woman can only be nulliparous, multiparous without a previous scar, or multiparous with at least one previous scar (previous obstetric record). A woman can only deliver by going into spontaneous labour, having labour induced, or delivered by Caesarean section before labour (course of pregnancy). Lastly, a pregnancy's gestational age is unique, provided an accepted method of calculation is agreed. All of the 5 obstetric concepts and their parameters fit the principles required for a classification system.[4]

Each of the 10 groups can and should be further subdivided when more detailed information about the groups is required. The indications for Caesarean section should be specifically defined within each group of women, because the definition and the management may vary in each group.

Table 2 The obstetric concepts and their parameters

Obstetric concept	Parameter
Category of pregnancy	Single cephalic pregnancy Single breech pregnancy Single oblique or transverse lie Multiple pregnancy
Previous obstetric record	Nulliparous Multiparous (without a uterine scar) Multiparous (with a uterine scar)
Course of labour and delivery	Spontaneous labour Induced labour Caesarean section before labour (Elective or emergency)
Gestation	Gestational age in completed weeks at time of delivery

Table 3 The 10 group classification, Stavanger, Norway 2001[17]

Groups	Overall Caesarean section (CS) rate (%) – 433/3959 (10.9%)			
	No. CS over total No. women in each group	Relative size of groups (%)	CS rate in each group (%)	Contribution made by each group to the overall CS rate of 10.9%
1. Nulliparous, single cephalic, ≥ 37 weeks, in spontaneous labour	56/1097	27.7 (1097/3959)	5.1 (56/1097)	1.4 (56/3959)
2. Nulliparous, single cephalic, ≥ 37 weeks, induced or CS before labour	63/274	6.9 (274/3959)	23.0 (63/274)	1.6 (63/3959)
3. Multiparous (excluding previous CS), single cephalic, ≥ 37 weeks, in spontaneous labour	14/1702	43.0 (1702/3959)	0.8 (14/1702)	0.4 (14/3959)
4. Multiparous (excluding previous CS), single cephalic, ≥ 37 weeks, induced or CS before labour	50/282	7.1 (282/3959)	17.7 (50/282)	1.3 (50/3959)
5. Previous CS, single cephalic, ≥ 37 weeks	79/190	4.8 (190/3959)	41.6 (79/190)	2.0 (79/3959)
6. All nulliparous breeches	55/67	1.7 (67/3959)	82.1 (55/67)	1.4 (55/3959)
7. All multiparous breeches (including previous CS)	36/57	1.4 (57/3959)	63.2 (36/57)	0.9 (36/3959)
8. All multiple pregnancies (including previous CS)	38/93	2.3 (93/3959)	40.9 (38/93)	1.0 (38/3959)
9. All abnormal lies (including previous CS)	10/10	0.3 (10/3959)	100 (10/10)	0.2 (10/3959)
10. All single cephalic, ≤ 36 weeks (including previous CS)	32/187	4.7 (187/3959)	17.1 (32/187)	0.8 (32/3959)

Therefore, assuming concern that a Caesarean section rate is too high, and also assuming that all the other childbirth outcome information required is available, then the 10 groups can be used in the assessment of any Caesarean section rate, and compared with other lower or higher Caesarean section rates either within the same delivery unit from previous years, or in other delivery units. This would reveal the groups of women with differences in the incidence of Caesarean sections and whether any advantages in other childbirth outcomes result. Why there is a difference in the number of Caesarean sections carried out will not be explained without further analysis, but a more logical and focused assessment will be possible.

The methodology using these concepts and their parameters to classify and audit Caesarean section rates has been successful in reducing the Caesarean section rate.[14] The audit cycle was used to identify and instigate changes in the management of labour in a specific group of woman, resulting in a safe and acceptable decrease in the Caesarean section rate. The 10-group classification is currently being used internationally,[17-19] and should provide helpful information in the assessment of Caesarean section rates.

Interpretation of Caesarean section rates using the 10 groups

Tables 1, 3 and 4, respectively, show the Caesarean section rates from Wycombe General Hospital, England, Stavanger Hospital, Norway,[17] and the total Caesarean section rate of England and Wales from the National Sentinel Caesarean Section Audit Report (NSCSA).[2] The 10 groups are presented as described in the original paper.[4] Only percentages are available from the NSCSA report, and the only other difference in Table 4 is the last column where, for the purpose of consistency, the percentage contribution to the overall Caesarean section rate made by each group adds up to the overall Caesarean section rate in the unit rather than to a total of 100% as described in the NSCSA.

The three tables show overall Caesarean section rates of 21%, 10.9% and 21.5%. In all 3 tables, groups 5,2 and 1 contribute most to the Caesarean section rate in that order. In each table, these groups contribute to at least half of the total Caesarean section rate. The difference between the tables is that the overall contribution of these groups is much bigger in Tables 1 and 4, accounting for most of the difference between the total Caesarean section rates. Clearly, the more Caesarean sections performed in groups 1 and 2 are likely to result in a larger group 5 in the future if those women have further pregnancies. If possible, unnecessary Caesarean sections in groups 1 and 2 should, therefore, be avoided. These three groups need to be studied in more detail if the overall Caesarean section rates in Tables 1 and 4 are going to be influenced.

Group 5 differs significantly not only in the size of the groups but also the Caesarean section rates within the groups. More information is required about group 5: in particular, the breakdown of how many women laboured spontaneously, how many were induced, and how many Caesarean sections were carried out before labour, including their indications.

Similar information is also required on group 2 on the number of inductions, the number of Caesarean sections carried out before labour, and their indications.

Lastly, the large variation in the Caesarean section rates between the different tables in group 1 is of concern: spontaneously labouring, nulliparous

Table 4 The 10 group classification, England and Wales, 2000[2]

Groups	Overall Caesarean section (CS) rate (%) – (21.5%)		
	No. CS over total No. women in each group		
	Relative size of groups (%)	CS rate in each group (%)	Contribution made by each group to the overall CS rate of 21.5%
1. Nulliparous, single cephalic, ≥ 37 weeks, in spontaneous labour	24.8	12.2	3.0
2. Nulliparous, single cephalic, ≥ 37 weeks, induced or CS before labour	10.8	34.6	3.8
3. Multiparous (excluding previous CS), single cephalic, ≥ 37 weeks, in spontaneous labour	33.0	3.1	1.0
4. Multiparous (excluding previous CS), single cephalic, ≥ 37 weeks, induced or CS before labour	10.7	18.1	2.0
5. Previous CS, single cephalic, ≥ 37 weeks	8.0	64.4	5.2
6. All nulliparous breeches	1.9	91.7	1.7
7. All multiparous breeches (including previous CS)	1.7	83.9	1.4
8. All multiple pregnancies (including previous CS)	1.5	59.5	1.0
9. All abnormal lies (including previous CS)	0.4	99.7	0.4
10. All single cephalic, ≤ 36 weeks (including previous CS)	5.8	33.0	1.9

women with a single cephalic pregnancy at term. Detailed information is required on the indications for Caesarean sections and the type of management carried out.

Further comparison between the tables shows differences in the relative sizes of groups 3, 4 and 10. This will contribute a small part to the difference in the overall Caesarean section rates, as relatively smaller sized groups 3 and 4 and a relatively larger group 10 will, in Tables 1 and 4, result in a slightly higher Caesarean section rate.

There is very little difference between the contributions in the three tables to the overall Caesarean section rate by groups 6–9 and, therefore, from the point of view of influencing the overall Caesarean section rate, these groups are not relevant.

In conclusion, if there is a concern about the higher Caesarean section rates in Tables 1 and 4, then the groups of women that deserve attention are 5,2 and 1. If information were available for the previous years for Tables 1 and 4, then obviously that would be helpful to explain how any changes in the Caesarean section rates may have occurred, especially in relation to other childbirth outcomes.

MATERNAL AND PERINATAL MORBIDITY AND MORTALITY

Within the data set, information on maternal and perinatal morbidity and mortality is required. The standardisation of information collection and classifications of these outcomes still requires a lot of work. Data on long-term outcome will be more difficult to collect accurately than short-term outcome, but will be necessary if we are to answer the question addressed in this chapter. This would require the establishment of local and national databases using the same definitions.

Just as collection of information on Caesarean section rates has been lacking, the same is true of information on maternal and perinatal morbidity and mortality on a continuous and statutory basis. The same principles of information collection need to be applied. At present, uncertainty continues about what information should be collected and there is no plan to collect information for the evaluation of long-term outcome.

MATERNAL SATISFACTION

Information on maternal satisfaction is a particular challenge; nevertheless, attempts have to be made to collect this information on a continuous and structured basis. This is a difficult area for standardised definitions and classification. Maternal satisfaction is best assessed by providing debriefing forms to all women who deliver in a unit.[20]

Maternal satisfaction is becoming one of the most significant childbirth outcomes.[21,22] At times, maternal satisfaction may unfortunately conflict with other targets set, such as a particular Caesarean section rate, making it both difficult and confusing for healthcare professionals. Healthcare professionals need to adapt their information collection and the setting of targets accordingly.

MEDICOLEGAL CASES AND COMPLAINTS

In the interpretation of any Caesarean section rate, the number of medicolegal cases should be recorded including those contested in court and settled out of court. In addition, any complaints related to the mode and timing of delivery should also be recorded. It has been suggested that the Caesarean section rate has risen as a direct result of the threat of litigation. This could be investigated by comparing information between countries with different cultures regarding litigation and complaints.

With individual awards for birth-related neurological handicap now exceeding £3 million in the UK, the effect of the threat of the litigation may indeed be real. The fear of being involved in a court case or a complaint may be partly responsible for obstetricians carrying out a Caesarean section with no definite medical indication but enough uncertainty present. The obstetrician may not be convinced that a court or an independent tribunal will retrospectively accept the situation of uncertainty and give fair consideration to the prospective professional decision made at the time. Society has become far less tolerant of poor outcomes generally, and the trend has continually been towards finding blame either with individuals or systems. The indications for Caesarean sections in these situations of uncertainty should be recorded as medical indications and the reasons given, but in addition some recognition of uncertainty of benefit should be recorded. The Caesarean sections that are carried out for this type of indication should be open to scrutiny and discussion amongst professionals.

AVAILABLE RESOURCES AND EXPERTISE

Information is required on the availability of relevant resources in a modern delivery unit, including the number of experienced staff, appropriate facilities, and equipment. In addition, staff satisfaction, recruitment and retention are all areas that need careful monitoring as directly or indirectly they may affect Caesarean section rates.

ACCEPTABILITY TO WOMEN

The responsibility for the current Caesarean section rate may no longer be exclusively that of professional healthcare workers. It may be time now to replace **natural** and **normal** as our criteria for practice in midwifery and obstetrics with **an open concept of the good**.[23] If this approach is adopted, it will not be the professionals who will decide what is good and what is bad, but instead, the informed and autonomous woman in pregnancy. Furthermore, what makes the professional health care practitioner **professional** is his or her knowledge of **means and consequences**, not his or her opinion about what is good or bad.[23]

Consequently, if Caesarean section rates are going to be influenced, the responsibility for Caesarean sections must first be clarified and agreed. Professional healthcare workers may be able to reduce a Caesarean section rate safely or keep the Caesarean section rate relatively low, but this would need to be accepted by women. The acceptability to women will depend on the quality of information, the clarity of argument and the trust they have in their carers.

Childbirth has always been an important issue within society which arouses strong feelings. These feelings need to be harnessed when deciding where responsibility lies for childbirth and how childbirth can be best cared for. Caesarean section rates can no longer be considered in isolation from other changes taking place within a society and differences between different countries.

In the UK, two major reports were published in the last 10 years which have had a significant influence on childbirth. *Changing Childbirth*[24] encouraged women to decide for themselves the type of care they would wish, the sort of professional they wish to carry it out, the place of delivery, and the degree of intervention. The Audit Commission, *First Class Delivery: Improving Maternity Services in England in Wales*,[25] announced that maternity services need to become more women-centred. Since these reports have been published, the number of women requesting Caesarean sections has increased. It is not clear whether the two are related. Other reports, internationally, have also encouraged patients to become more involved in their treatment,[26] interestingly in countries with high Caesarean section rates.[27]

The National Sentinel Caesarean Section Audit (NSCSA)[2] carried out recently in the UK confirmed that a significant proportion of women wanted more information on the risks and benefits of Caesarean sections. If such information is available in a clear and concise form, then it is likely that healthcare professionals and women would agree in most cases about the most appropriate mode of delivery. The NSCSA also confirmed previous studies that a significant number of women request delivery by Caesarean section. All the studies suffer from lack of definition of the term 'maternal request', but a significant number of women do not accept professional advice that a Caesarean section is not necessary on medical grounds.

The incidence of Caesarean section for maternal request varies, and in some delivery units does not arise. Some units do not acknowledge maternal request as an indication for Caesarean section and either do not agree to carry out the Caesarean section, or record an alternative pseudomedical indication for the Caesarean section. Whether or not a Caesarean section should be carried out on request is a controversial issue.[28,29] Women may request Caesarean sections for a number of reasons and, although they may not all be medically indicated, many of the requests are understandable. A consensus regarding the justification of Caesarean section for maternal request is unlikely to be reached, but the indication needs to be recognised, accepted, formally defined and recorded. The logical approach is to introduce a formal process to deal with the issue, and record the reasons why women are requesting Caesarean sections. Once the reasons why women request Caesarean sections have been identified and the necessary information is available, then it should be possible to decide whether the requests can be justified, and whether some of the requests can be avoided. In addition, the complications from Caesarean sections carried out for maternal request should be recorded.

The ethical, legal and economic implications of carrying out Caesarean sections for maternal request are significant.[30–34] If maternal request for Caesarean section is accepted as an indication, then all indications for Caesarean section will need to be divided into two main categories. First, those Caesarean sections that are carried out for medical reasons, where on balance the obstetrician advises the patient that a Caesarean section is the most appropriate method of delivery. Second, those where the women pre-empt the obstetrician, by requesting a Caesarean section when on balance the obstetrician would advise an attempt to deliver vaginally.

From a professional point of view, this differentiation of indications for Caesarean sections would be of great importance. Problems will arise in the differentiation because, undoubtedly, obstetricians' opinions will differ. This should not prevent obstetricians from attempting to differentiate between the two types of indication. This difference of opinion between obstetricians should become less, provided the information available on the short- and long-term outcome of Caesarean sections improves. The relative incidences of Caesarean section for medical indications and for maternal request will help to delineate the responsibility for, and the appropriateness of, different Caesarean section rates. An indication for Caesarean section as a maternal request today, with change in practice and outcomes from Caesarean sections, may become a medical indication in the future.

SAFE IMPLEMENTATION

In the author's view, provided the first two criteria, justification and acceptability to women, are met, the 10 groups and their sub-groups can be used to instigate specific changes and monitor any changes. However, the background organisation within which changes are made on the labour ward is crucial.

The labour ward audit cycle (Fig. 1) summarises the auditing of labour ward events and outcome: classifying and assessing them, modification of management and continuation of auditing results. The principles of labour ward audit have been described elsewhere in detail[20] and need to be fully understood and implemented before any change of practice is attempted and especially before attempting the reduction of a Caesarean section rate. Active participation in collecting the information should be part of the responsibility of all the professionals working on the labour ward. After classification of the crude data, the information needs to be disseminated among the professionals involved in labour and delivery. Assessment of management at some stage involves setting targets of care that are thought to be desirable. One of those targets will be an appropriate Caesarean section rate, but this cannot be considered in isolation from other childbirth outcomes. In addition, the available resources and expertise, as well as staff satisfaction need to be taken into account when setting targets.

To set targets and assess management, regular multidisciplinary meetings are required. No improvements to perinatal care can take place until we become multidisciplinary, and that will mean significant cultural changes for all the

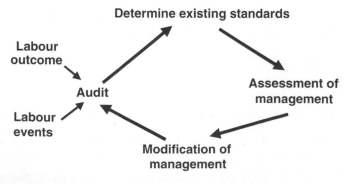

Fig. 1 The labour ward audit cycle.

professionals involved. These meetings require a mutual respect for the different professional points of view, which should be based on knowledge of quality information. This information must include both local outcome and published data. A daily morning meeting lasting approximately 30 min is most appropriate, attended, supported and led by senior midwifery and medical staff, with all staff attending on a regular basis. The relevant events in the previous 24 h in the labour ward should be discussed, and present on-going issues regarding the management of labour. The success of these meetings depends on a good information system within the department and adequate preparation for each meeting. The return for this commitment by all the staff is good team-work and communication in the department. Detailed written guidelines in the management of labour and delivery may be helpful as an adjunct in certain units, but must not replace the daily morning meetings with continuous education and discussion.

Implementing and maintaining high standards of care will depend on the general organisation of the labour ward, a well-trained, permanent midwifery staff supported by direct consultant involvement.

Finally, the professional responsible for the labour ward on a multidisciplinary basis should be responsible for the organisation and running of the daily meetings and given the appropriate authority and support.

Key points for clinical practice

- Information needs to be clinically relevant, carefully defined, accurately collected, timely and available.

- Caesarean sections should be audited using the obstetrical concepts and their parameters and standardised indications for inductions and Caesarean sections.

- Monthly critical analysis of the 10 groups is required including comparison with previous months in the same units and also in other units, subdividing the 10 groups for more detailed analysis as appropriate.

- To implement change, a good information system is required with daily multidisciplinary meetings.

- Senior midwifery and medical leadership is essential with commitment from all staff to the meetings.

- Changes to management of labour are made as appropriate, with daily, continuous critical assessment.

References

1. Robson MS. Can we reduce the Caesarean section rate? *Baillière's Clin Obstet Gynaecol* 2001; **15**: 179–194.
2. Thomas J, Paranjothy S and The Royal College of Obstetricians and Gynaecologists, Clinical Effectiveness Support Unit. *The National Sentinel Caesarean Section Audit Report.* London: RCOG Press, 2001.
3. Sachs BP, Kobelin C, Castro MA, Frigoletto F. The risks of lowering the Cesarean-delivery rate. *N Engl J Med* 1999; **340**: 54–57.

4. Robson MS. Classification of Caesarean sections. *Fetal Matern Med Rev* 2001; **12**: 23–39.
5. Anderson GM, Lomas J. Determinants of the increasing Cesarean birth rate. *N Engl J Med* 1984; **311**: 887–892.
6. Steer P. Caesarean section: an evolving procedure? *Br J Obstet Gynaecol* 1998; **105**: 1052–1055.
7. MacArthur C, Bick DE, Keighley MR. Faecal incontinence after childbirth. *Br J Obstet Gynaecol* 1997; **104**: 46–50.
8. Sultan AH, Kamm MA, Hudson CN, Thomas JM, Bartram CI. Anal sphincter disruption during vaginal delivery. *N Engl J Med* 1993; **329**: 1906–1911.
9. Viktrup L, Lose G, Rolff M, Barfoed K. The symptoms of stress incontinence caused by pregnancy or delivery in primiparas. *Obstet Gynecol* 1992; **79**: 945–949.
10. Glazener C. Sexual function after childbirth: women's experiences, persistent morbidity and lack of professional recognition. *Br J Obstet Gynaecol* 1997; **104**: 330–335.
11. Paterson-Brown S. Should doctors perform an elective Caesarean section on request? Yes, as long as the woman is fully informed. *BMJ* 1998; **317**: 462–463.
12. Sultan AH, Stanton SL. Preserving the pelvic floor and perineum during childbirth – elective Caesarean section? *Br J Obstet Gynaecol* 1996; **103**: 731–734.
13. Feldman GB, Freiman JA. Prophylactic Cesarean section at term? *N Engl J Med* 1985; **312**: 1264–1267.
14. Robson MS, Scudamore IW, Walsh SM. Using the medical audit cycle to reduce Cesarean section rates. *Am J Obstet Gynecol* 1996; **174**: 199–205.
15. Notzon FC, Cnattingius S, Bergsjø P *et al.* Cesarean section delivery in the 1980s: international comparison by indication. *Am J Obstet Gynecol* 1994; **170**: 495–504.
16. Cleary R, Beard RW, Chapple J *et al.* The standard primipara as a basis for inter-unit comparisons of maternity care. *Br J Obstet Gynaecol* 1996; **103**: 223–229.
17. Gjessing L. <http://www.gjessing.no/06_KVALRING_PUBL/QIPO_2001/ KK_RING_YEARALL_C3_ROBSON_.htm> Accessed on 15/09/2002.
18. <http://www.foedsels-audit.suite.dk/> Accessed on 15/09/2002.
19. The National Maternity Hospital, Dublin, Ireland. *Annual Clinical Report*. Dublin: The National Maternity Hospital, 2000; 98–100.
20. Robson MS. Labour ward audit. In: Creasy R. (ed) *Management of Labour and Delivery*. Oxford: Blackwell, 1997; 559–570.
21. Mould TAJ, Chong S, Spencer JAD, Gallivan S. Women's involvement with the decision preceding their Caesarean section and their degree of satisfaction. *Br J Obstet Gynaecol* 1996; **103**: 1074–1077.
22. Graham WJ, Hundley V, McCheyne AL, Hall MH, Gurney E, Milne J. An investigation of women's involvement in the decision to deliver by Caesarean section. *Br J Obstet Gynaecol* 1999; **106**: 213–220.
23. Wackerhausen S. What is natural? Deciding what to do and not to do in medicine and health care. *Br J Obstet Gynaecol* 1999; **106**: 1109–1112.
24. Department of Health. *Changing Childbirth: The Report of the Expert Maternity Group*. London: HMSO, 1993.
25. Audit Commission. First Class Delivery: Improving Maternity Services in England in Wales. Abingdon: Audit Commission Publications, 1997.
26. Legge Reginale n.23 2/6/1992: diritti della partoriente e del bambino ospedalizzato. Boll Uff Reg 1992; **32**: 2155–2159.
27. Parazzini F, Pirotta N, La Vecchia C, Fedele L. Determinants of Caesarean section rates in Italy. Br J Obstet Gynaecol 1992; **99**: 203–206.
28. Amu O, Rajendran S, Bolaji I. Should doctors perform an elective Caesarean section on request? Maternal choice alone should not determine method of delivery. BMJ 1998; **317**: 463–465.
29. Showalter E, Griffin A. Commentary: all women should have a choice. *BMJ* 1999; **319**: 1401.
30. Anon. Is there a legal right to choose a Caesarean section? *Br J Midwifery* 1999; **7**: 515–518.
31. Goldbeck-Wood S. Women's autonomy in childbirth. *BMJ* 1997; **314**: 1143–1144.
32. MacKenzie IZ. Should women who elect to have Caesarean sections pay for them [letter]? *BMJ* 1999; **318**: 1070.
33. Bewley S, Cockburn J. I. The unethics of 'request' Caesarean section. *Br J Obstet Gynaecol* 2002; **109**: 593–596.
34. Bewley S, Cockburn J. II. The unfacts of 'request' Caesarean section. *Br J Obstet Gynaecol* 2002; **109**: 597–605.

Deirdre J. Murphy

7

Maternal and neonatal morbidity following operative delivery in the second stage of labour

Recent media and medical interest has focused on the rising Caesarean section rate, and in particular, whether women should be able to choose elective Caesarean section as a preferred mode of delivery. This has distracted us from addressing the concerns of labouring women. The fact remains that the majority of women still aim for spontaneous vaginal delivery and are supported in their endeavours by the majority of obstetricians. Women who experience arrested progress in the second stage of labour may be presented with an apparent conflict between maternal and neonatal well-being. The careful obstetrician is aiming for the lowest morbidity for both mother and baby and faces a difficult choice between a potentially complex instrumental vaginal delivery and Caesarean section at full dilatation, each with inherent risks. Obstetricians have strong views about the management of women with arrested progress in the second stage, which has so far limited randomised controlled trials addressing this issue. Nonetheless, it is vital that informed decisions are made, based on the best available evidence rather than solely on the professional carer's opinion. It is also essential that full consideration be given to short- and long-term consequences of the chosen mode of operative delivery as well as the implications for future reproductive and delivery outcomes.

EPIDEMIOLOGY OF OPERATIVE DELIVERY

There has been a steady decrease in the proportion of women achieving spontaneous vaginal delivery in industrialised countries throughout the world.[1] This is reflected in a dramatic rise in rates of operative delivery. Rates of Caesarean section in North America exceeded 25% in the last decade and have now stabilised below 25%. A recent evaluation of Caesarean delivery by a task force for the American College of Obstetricians and Gynecologists

Deirdre J. Murphy MB BCh BAO DipEpidem MD MRCOG, Professor of Obstetrics and Gynaecology, Ninewells Hospital and Medical School, Dundee DD1 9SY, UK

reported that first-time mothers delivering a term singleton cephalic fetus and women with a previous Caesarean section account for two-thirds of all Caesarean deliveries in the US.[2] Most of the dramatic variation in Caesarean delivery rates occurred in these two groups. Improved training in operative vaginal delivery has been recommended and it was suggested that safe use of these techniques may help reduce the Caesarean delivery rate.[2]

The National Sentinel Caesarean Section audit provided detailed information on operative delivery rates for England, Wales and Northern Ireland.[1] The Caesarean section rate in England was 21.3% with rates of 24.2% and 23.9% in Wales and Northern Ireland, respectively. This compares with a Caesarean section rate of 12% in Norway. Operative vaginal delivery rates ranged from 10–12% and have remained constant. The majority of instrumental deliveries were by forceps in 1980 with 60–70% performed by ventouse in 2000–2001.[1] Of note, ventouse delivery has been associated with a higher failure rate and, therefore, greater likelihood of recourse to Caesarean section.[3]

The primary Caesarean section rate (first Caesarean section in women of any parity) for the audit was 17% overall.[1] The main indications were presumed fetal compromise, failure to progress and breech presentation. The repeat Caesarean section rate was 67% in England, 66% in Wales and 76% in Northern Ireland. The majority of women have a singleton pregnancy with a cephalic presentation born at term. Although the Caesarean section rate for these women was 17%, as the largest clinical group in the population they contribute 70% to the overall Caesarean section rate. Clearly, the management of a first labour will have a major impact on the overall Caesarean section rate for any delivery unit. The authors report dramatic regional variation in Caesarean section rates with a rate of 19% in the South West of England compared to a rate of 24% in London. These differences cannot be explained by demographic differences in the populations alone.

In stark contrast, the observed rate of Caesarean section in West Africa was 1.3% with a suggested range of 3.6–6.5% for maternal indications alone.[4] These estimates fall well below the World Health Organization's recommendation of a 10–15% Caesarean section rate set to achieve optimal maternal and perinatal safety. This report suggests that there is restricted access to appropriate obstetric care in non-industrialised countries for maternal indications that are major determinants of serious maternal morbidity and mortality.

It is more difficult to establish rates of Caesarean section in the second stage of labour. In a recent prospective cohort study of women in the South West of England, 4% of the total population were transferred to theatre for operative delivery in the second stage of labour and just over half of these women were delivered by Caesarean section.[3] This overall rate is similar to the rate of breech presentation at term. The women delivered by instrumental vaginal delivery reflect the severe end of the spectrum of operative difficulty as uncomplicated instrumental deliveries are usually performed in the delivery room. A North American review of operative vaginal delivery in the year 2000 suggested that operative deliveries involving rotation of more than 45° were likely to be abandoned. This has been reflected in a survey of obstetric fellows of the American College of Obstetricians and Gynecologists which showed that over half have abandoned mid-cavity assisted vaginal delivery in favour of

Caesarean section.[5] Clearly, there are concerns about maternal and infant safety in relation to complex instrumental vaginal delivery. The potential for morbidity following operative delivery in the second stage of labour needs to be addressed in the context of an ever rising Caesarean section rate and escalating claims of negligence in relation to intrapartum care.

MATERNAL MORBIDITY

For many women, operative delivery is not planned or even considered and is a particularly disappointing result when it is the outcome of a long and difficult second stage of labour. There is an increased risk of maternal morbidity following operative delivery that may result in unplanned hospital admission and a protracted period of recovery. The complications that arise may have their origin in the indication for assisted delivery or may result from the procedure itself. It is important to consider not only the potential for long-term complications due to genital tract trauma and scar tissue formation, but also the implications for future pregnancies and delivery. The psychological and psychosexual impact of operative delivery have received little attention to date.

EARLY MORBIDITY

Currently, we have a dearth of high quality evidence on which to base decisions relating to difficult delivery in the second stage of labour. Debate is on-going on the relative merits and hazards of ventouse and forceps delivery. A systematic review reported that use of the vacuum extractor (ventouse) was associated with significantly less maternal trauma (odds ratio, 0.41; 95% CI, 0.33–0.50) and with more completed deliveries (odds ratio, 1.69; 95% CI, 1.31–2.19) than forceps delivery.[6] However, trial of forceps was more likely to result in completed vaginal delivery than attempted ventouse in a study of women transferred to theatre for arrested progress in the second stage of labour (63% *versus* 48%, $P < 0.01$).[3] In a recent US study, forceps delivery increased overall maternal complications with higher rates of postpartum infection, cervical laceration and prolonged hospital stay than for women delivered by ventouse.[7] These findings are reflected in a marked increase in the use of ventouse for vaginal instrumental delivery over the past two decades.[1]

For rotational delivery, manual rotation, rotational ventouse and Caesarean section have overtaken Kielland's forceps in popularity.[3] However, the introduction of a new vacuum extraction device, the Kiwi Omnicup, has expanded the available options for rotational delivery; Vacca has reported a 98% success rate for 18 non-rotational and 32 rotational vacuum assisted deliveries with a very low rate of morbidity.[8] The Kiwi Omnicup may provide an efficient and safe instrument for assisted rotational vaginal delivery, but outcomes need to be evaluated in the hands of less-experienced obstetricians.

In practice, true mid-cavity arrest in the second stage of labour presents the obstetrician with a choice between difficult instrumental vaginal delivery and Caesarean section at full dilatation. There has been inconsistency in the reported early maternal morbidity when comparing these delivery options. This may reflect the retrospective design of most studies and the methodological biases inherent with such work. In a review of the maternal and fetal outcome of failed instrumental delivery compared to proceeding directly to Caesarean section in the second stage of labour, Revah *et al.*[9] found no increased morbidity for the mother in a setting where Caesarean section could follow promptly. Older studies comparing mid-cavity forceps with Caesarean section found a significant increase in maternal morbidity in the Caesarean section group with longer hospital stays and more frequent maternal haemorrhage and infection.

In a prospective cohort study of women transferred to theatre for second stage arrest, Caesarean section was associated with an increased risk of major haemorrhage (adjusted odds ratio, 2.8; 95% CI, 1.1–7.6) and prolonged hospital stay (odds ratio, 3.5; 95% CI, 1.6–7.6).[3] However, Caesarean delivery (odds ratio, 0.63; 95% CI, 0.38–1.00) and major haemorrhage were less likely with an experienced obstetrician (odds ratio, 0.5; 95% CI, 0.3–0.9). High rates of third and fourth degree tears are reported following instrumental vaginal delivery. The comparable morbidity at Caesarean section relates to extension of the uterine incision into the cervix, vagina or broad ligaments. Extension of the uterine incision at full dilatation has been reported in up to 35% of cases,[10] and has been associated with an increased risk of Caesarean hysterectomy and febrile morbidity. Long-term follow-up will determine whether this results in subsequent difficult deliveries or an increased risk of uterine rupture.

Clearly, choice of operative delivery in the second stage of labour presents a difficult risk/benefit dilemma. Caesarean section at full dilatation with anhydramnios and an engaged fetal head is a difficult procedure. This is reflected in high rates of major obstetric haemorrhage, extension of the uterine incision and prolonged hospital admission. These risks must be balanced with the potential for pelvic floor trauma following instrumental vaginal delivery.

PELVIC FLOOR MORBIDITY

Instrumental vaginal delivery is associated with increased pelvic floor morbidity, but comparisons between ventouse and forceps remain controversial. Forceps delivery incurred a higher risk of third-degree laceration than ventouse in two population-based studies (odds ratio, 1.94; 95% CI, 1.30–2.89 and odds ratio, 3.33; 95% CI, 2.97–3.74, respectively).[11,12] In another study, vacuum delivery (odds ratio, 2.30; 95% CI, 2.21–2.40) presented a greater risk of sphincter laceration than forceps delivery (odds ratio, 1.45- 95% CI, 1.37–1.52).[13] There was no difference in rates of urinary and bowel dysfunction at 5-year follow-up of a randomised controlled study comparing forceps and ventouse delivery.[14] However, symptoms of dysfunction were very prevalent with 47% of women reporting urinary incontinence of varying severity and 44% bowel habit urgency. In a survey of Australian adults, pelvic floor dysfunction (urinary and faecal incontinence) was significantly associated with at least one instrumental delivery (odds ratio, 4.3; 95% CI, 2.8–6.6) which suggests that delivery-related morbidity has both short- and long-term health implications.[15]

Historically, episiotomy has been considered an inherent part of forceps delivery. With the increasing popularity of ventouse delivery, there has been a tendency to avoid episiotomy with the aim to achieve instrumental delivery with an intact perineum. Such practice has not been exposed to rigorous evaluation to date. The role of episiotomy in preventing third and fourth degree tears is controversial. A multicentre, international survey of women at 3 months after delivery found no association between faecal incontinence and duration of second stage labour or use of episiotomy.[11] In contrast, authors of a large population-based study in The Netherlands found that mediolateral episiotomy protected strongly against the occurrence of third degree perineal ruptures (odds ratio, 0.21; 95% CI, 0.20–0.23) and thus may serve as a primary method of prevention of faecal incontinence.[12] To confuse matters further, Handa *et al.* report that among two million Californian women episiotomy decreased the likelihood of third-degree lacerations (odds ratio, 0.81; 95% CI, 0.78–0.85) but increased the risk of fourth-degree lacerations (odds ratio, 1.12; 95% CI, 1.05–1.19).[13] In a US study of operative vaginal deliveries, forceps delivery without episiotomy was not associated with a difference in the occurrence of significant perineal trauma (RR, 1.2; 95% CI, 0.8–1.9).[16] Among vacuum extraction deliveries, an increased rate of trauma was noted when episiotomy was used (RR, 3.7; 95% CI, 1.2–1.2). Cultural differences are important, however, as midline episiotomy is favoured in the US and has been associated with increased anorectal morbidity while mediolateral episiotomy is preferred in Europe.

PSYCHOLOGICAL MORBIDITY

A previous delivery experience can have important implications for future pregnancies, not least whether a woman would contemplate another pregnancy. Fear of childbirth has been reported in up to 26% of women at 5 years following either instrumental vaginal delivery or Caesarean section compared with 10% following spontaneous vaginal delivery.[17] This contrasts with the findings of a survey of primigravidae who described similar experiences of forceps and unassisted deliveries but found delivery by Caesarean section to be less difficult, but more distressing, than either type of vaginal delivery.[18] A randomised controlled trial was conducted in Australia to assess the effectiveness of a midwife-led debriefing session during the postpartum hospital stay in reducing maternal depression among women giving birth by Caesarean section, forceps or ventouse extraction.[19] Midwife-led debriefing was ineffective in reducing maternal morbidity at 6 months' postpartum and the authors commented that the possibility that debriefing contributed to emotional health problems for some women could not be excluded. Further research is required to establish an optimal approach to helping women come to terms with the fear, distress and depression that can result from operative delivery.

FUTURE REPRODUCTIVE OUTCOME

Long-term fertility consequences are recognised following operative deliveries. Primiparous women who delivered by Caesarean section have been shown to have fewer children and more difficulty conceiving than controls.[20] An increased risk of voluntary and involuntary infertility following primary Caesarean section and to some extent vaginal instrumental delivery has also been reported.[17] A recent population-based cohort study addressed the time to conception for women who chose to have a further pregnancy.[21] A history of previous Caesarean section was associated with an increased risk of taking more than 1 year to conceive from the time of planning a pregnancy (odds ratio, 1.74; 95% CI, 1.26–2.40). Of note, the risk remained significant after controlling for important potential confounding factors such as maternal and paternal age at conception, cohabitation duration, oral contraceptive pill use, cigarette exposure, educational level, ethnicity, parity, change of partner and maternal body mass index. A further study reports equal rates of subsequent childbearing for primigravidae who experienced instrumental delivery for mid-cavity arrest and primigravidae who had spontaneous vaginal deliveries.[22]

There appears to be an association between operative delivery and subsequent voluntary and involuntary infertility, particularly following Caesarean section. Further quantitative and qualitative studies are required to confirm whether these associations are causal and to explore potential aetiological factors.

FUTURE DELIVERY OUTCOME

The mode of delivery for arrested progress in the second stage of labour may have important implications for future mode of delivery. Women who have experienced a previous Caesarean section at full dilatation generate anxiety in subsequent labours relating to the risk of further emergency Caesarean section and potential uterine rupture.[23] Mid-cavity and rotational instrumental vaginal deliveries have become unpopular in the US and are increasingly abandoned in favour of Caesarean section.[5] This may be a short-sighted view, however, if one fails to consider the outcome of future deliveries in the assessment of overall morbidity. An assisted vaginal delivery in an earlier pregnancy may increase the likelihood of future uncomplicated spontaneous vaginal deliveries. In a follow-up study of primigravidae who required mid-cavity instrumental delivery, more than 75% achieved a spontaneous vaginal delivery with heavier babies in the second pregnancy and very low overall rates of birth trauma or asphyxia.[22]

One of the principal arguments for proceeding to elective Caesarean section after a previous instrumental vaginal delivery is to avoid cumulative pelvic floor injury and, in particular, the potential for anal incontinence in women with occult and repaired anal sphincter injuries. Increased symptoms of urinary and faecal incontinence are associated with instrumental vaginal delivery.[15] Subsequent vaginal deliveries have been shown to increase the risk of anal incontinence among women with a previously diagnosed sphincter defect.[24] However, careful selection of women eligible for future vaginal delivery may help to alleviate concern. Of 45 pregnant women with a previous third-degree tear referred to a specialised perineal clinic for determination of future mode of delivery, 4 had a high symptom score and were delivered by elective Caesarean section and the remaining 41 (91%) opted for trial of vaginal delivery and all had spontaneous vaginal deliveries.[25] Women's satisfaction with the subsequent delivery experience remains to be evaluated.

NEONATAL MORBIDITY

The neonatal outcome is critical to the debate on optimal mode of operative delivery when complications arise in the second stage of labour. The need for speed may compete with concerns about neonatal trauma particularly where there are features of potential fetal compromise. The operator's expertise may ultimately determine the preferred mode of delivery, but each obstetrician should have the necessary skills to deliver the baby by the swiftest and safest means according to the individual circumstances.

CONDITION AT BIRTH

A British study conducted in the late 1970s examined the neonatal morbidity and mortality associated with Kielland's forceps delivery.[26] The authors reported a neonatal mortality rate of 34.9 per 1000 births, birth trauma in 15% of the survivors and abnormal neurological behaviour in 23% of the neonates which was not attributable to birth asphyxia alone. Such levels of neonatal morbidity and mortality are unacceptable in modern obstetrical practice and have been reflected in less frequent use of Kielland's forceps and only in the hands of experienced operators and in carefully selected cases. The current management of mid-cavity arrest more frequently involves manual rotation and forceps, non-rotational traction forceps, ventouse extraction and Caesarean section. The neonatal morbidity related to operative delivery needs to be evaluated where: (i) vaginal delivery is successfully achieved; (ii) Caesarean section is undertaken following failure of attempted instrumental vaginal delivery; and (iii) delivery is by immediate Caesarean section.

In a systematic review of trials comparing vacuum extraction with forceps delivery, Johanson and Menon reported that use of the vacuum extractor was associated with an increase in neonatal cephalhaematoma and retinal haemorrhages.[7] Despite this finding, the vacuum extractor has become the instrument of choice in the interest of minimizing maternal morbidity. If speed is of the essence, particularly in the presence of suspected fetal hypoxia, then forceps has been suggested as the instrument of choice. A prospective analysis of 225 women requiring instrumental delivery described a mean decision to delivery interval of 23.3 min (SD 14.3 min) for forceps procedures and 29.2 min (SD 13.2 min) for ventouse ($P = 0.04$).[27] Use of forceps was found to result in a quicker birth than use of ventouse without any compromise to the condition of the baby and with similar rates of perineal trauma.

To date, there has been inconsistency in the reported early neonatal morbidity when comparing instrumental vaginal delivery with Caesarean section for mid-cavity arrest. Older, retrospective studies found little difference in short-term neonatal morbidity and re-assuringly the study by Revah et al.[10] found no increase in neonatal morbidity among women who had a failed instrumental delivery in a setting where Caesarean section could follow promptly. In a prospective cohort study of women transferred to theatre in the second stage of labour, delivery by Caesarean section was associated with an increased risk of admission to the special care baby unit (SCBU) compared to instrumental vaginal delivery (odds ratio, 2.6; 95% CI, 1.2–6.0).[3] Of note, there were equal rates of ominous fetal heart rate tracings in the two groups. The greater risk of admission to SCBU following Caesarean section did not appear to be the result of a selective decision based on pre-existing fetal compromise, but may reflect the decision to delivery interval, which is frequently longer for a Caesarean section. However, neonatal trauma was significantly less common following Caesarean delivery compared to instrumental vaginal delivery (odds ratio, 0.4; 95% CI, 0.2–0.7). In the majority of cases, this represented facial and scalp bruising; however, there was one facial laceration in each group, and a fractured clavicle and 6 cases of brachial plexus injury in the vaginal delivery group. A low umbilical artery pH was more frequently recorded following failed instrumental delivery, but there was no increase in admissions to SCBU. Trauma was significantly more likely following failed instrumental delivery than immediate Caesarean section ($P = 0.03$), but was still less common than following successful instrumental delivery. This finding suggests that traumatic delivery could be reduced with careful selection of cases.

The safest, quickest mode of delivery needs to be the priority where there is evidence of fetal compromise and this may mean instrumental delivery in experienced hands. However, instrumental vaginal delivery is likely to incur an increased risk of birth trauma that is avoided by immediate recourse to Caesarean section.

DEVELOPMENTAL OUTCOME

Concerns about early morbidity are quickly replaced by concerns about survival and long-term neurological disability in situations where the baby is born in poor condition. This can occur following either instrumental vaginal delivery or Caesarean section and may result from the indication for emergency operative delivery and/or the procedure itself. Maternal fever, which is increased with long labour and instrumental delivery, has been strongly associated with neonatal encephalopathy (odds ratio, 10.8; 95% CI, 4.0–29.3).[28] Badawi et al. have reported an increased risk of neonatal encephalopathy following both instrumental vaginal delivery and emergency Caesarean section in a large Australian population-based study (odds ratio, 2.3; 95% CI, 1.2–4.7) and (odds ratio, 2.2; 95% CI, 1.0–4.6), respectively.[29] Moderate and severe neonatal encephalopathy are strongly associated with cerebral palsy and death. The use of sequential instruments particularly ventouse and forceps has been associated with scalp trauma, intracranial haemorrhage and neonatal death.[30]

Clearly, the choice and conduct of operative delivery in the second stage of labour may have far-reaching consequences. It is important that studies addressing morbidity evaluate long-term neurodevelopmental outcome as neurological, cognitive and social disability may not be apparent for some years.

CONCLUSIONS

Operative delivery in the second stage of labour continues to pose a challenge for the obstetrician. There is a balance to achieve between maternal and neonatal well-being and early and long-term morbidity. Obstetricians should aim to deliver by the safest and most appropriate mode within their expertise. A management approach that can only offer Caesarean section for complications in the second stage of labour may prove limiting and short-sighted. We are gaining increasing knowledge about long-term health implications of operative delivery for both mother and baby. The influence of obstetric management in such cases needs further evaluation in terms of maternal psychological morbidity, future subfertility both voluntary and involuntary, and the delivery outcome of future pregnancies.

Key points for clinical practice

- Currently, one in every three pregnant women in the UK experiences operative delivery.

- The vacuum extractor is preferred to forceps delivery in the interest of minimising maternal perineal trauma, but is associated with higher rates of neonatal trauma.

- An increasing proportion of deliveries for mid-cavity arrest and malrotation are undertaken by Caesarean section with a loss of expertise in complex instrumental vaginal delivery.

- Caesarean section in the second stage of labour is associated with higher rates of major obstetric haemorrhage, prolonged maternal hospital admission and more frequent neonatal admission for special care than instrumental vaginal delivery.

- Instrumental vaginal delivery is associated with a greater risk of pelvic floor trauma and subsequent urinary and bowel incontinence than Caesarean section.

- There is an increased risk of voluntary and involuntary subfertility following delivery by Caesarean section.

- Instrumental vaginal delivery and failed instrumental vaginal delivery are associated with higher rates of neonatal trauma than Caesarean section. This is a particular problem with the use of sequential instruments.

- Obstetricians should aim to deliver by the safest and most appropriate mode within their expertise balancing the risks of maternal and neonatal morbidity. This may be an indication for complex instrumental vaginal delivery in experienced hands.

References

1. Thomas J, Paranjothy S, The Royal College of Obstetricians and Gynaecologists Clinical Effectiveness Support Unit. *National Sentinel Caesarean Section Audit Report*. London: RCOG Press, 2001.
2. American College of Obstetricians and Gynecologists. *Evaluation of Cesarean Delivery*. Washington, DC: ACOG, 2000.
3. Murphy DJ, Liebling RE, Verity L, Swingler R, Patel R. Cohort study of the early maternal and neonatal morbidity associated with operative delivery in the second stage of labour. *Lancet* 2001; **358**: 1203–1207.
4. Dumont A, de Bernis L, Bouvier-Colle M-H, Breart G, for the MOMA Study Group. Caesarean section rate for maternal indication in sub-Saharan Africa: a systematic review. *Lancet* 2001; **358**: 1328–1334.
5. Bofill JA, Rust OA, Perry KG, Roberts WE, Martin RW, Morrison JC. Operative vaginal delivery: a survey of fellows of ACOG. *Obstet Gynecol* 1996; **88**: 1007–1010.
6. Johanson RB, Menon BK. Vacuum extraction versus forceps for assisted vaginal delivery. *Cochrane Database Syst Rev* 2000; (2): CD000224.
7. Kabiru WN, Jamieson D, Graves W, Lindsay M. Trends in operative vaginal delivery rates and associated maternal complication rates in an inner-city hospital. *Am J Obstet Gynecol* 2001; **184**: 1112–1114.

8. Vacca A. Operative vaginal delivery: clinical appraisal of a new vacuum extraction device. *Aust NZ J Obstet Gynaecol* 2001; **41**: 156–160.

9. Revah A, Ezra Y, Farine D, Ritchie K. Failed trial of vacuum or forceps – maternal and fetal outcome. *Am J Obstet Gynecol* 1997; **176**: 200–204.

10. Rodriguez AI, Porter KB, O'Brien WF. Blunt versus sharp expansion of the uterine incision in low-segment transverse Cesarean section. *Am J Obstet Gynecol* 1994; **171**: 1022–1025.

11. MacArthur C, Glazener CMA, Wilson PD *et al*. Obstetric practice and faecal incontinence three months after delivery. *Br J Obstet Gynaecol* 2001; **108**: 678–683.

12. De Leeuw JW, Struijk PC, Vierhout ME, Wallenburg HCS. Risk factors for third degree perineal ruptures during delivery. *Br J Obstet Gynaecol* 2001; **108**: 383–387.

13. Handa VL, Danielsen BH, Gilbert WM. Obstetric anal sphincter lacerations. *Obstet Gynecol* 2001; **98**: 225–230.

14. Johanson RB, Heycock E, Carter J, Sultan AH, Walklate K, Jones PW. Maternal and child health after assisted vaginal delivery: five-year follow up of a randomised controlled study comparing forceps and ventouse. *Br J Obstet Gynaecol* 1999; **106**: 544–549.

15. MacLennan AH, Taylor AW, Wilson DH, Wilson D. The prevalence of pelvic floor disorders and their relationship to gender, age, parity and mode of delivery. *Br J Obstet Gynaecol* 2000; **107**: 1460–1470.

16. Robinson JN, Norwitz ER, Cohen AP, McElrath TF, Lieberman ES. Episiotomy, operative vaginal delivery, and significant perineal trauma in nulliparous women. *Am J Obstet Gynecol* 1999; **181**: 1180–1184.

17. Jolly J, Walker J, Bhabra K. Subsequent obstetric performance related to primary mode of delivery. *Br J Obstet Gynaecol* 1999; **106**: 227–232.

18. Salmon P, Drew NC. Multidimensional assessment of women's experience of childbirth: relationship to obstetric procedure, antenatal preparation and obstetric history. *J Psychosom Res* 1992; **36**: 317–327.

19. Small R, Lumley J, Donohue L, Potter A, Waldenstrom U. Randomised controlled trial of midwife led debriefing to reduce maternal depression after operative childbirth. *BMJ* 2000; **321**: 1043–1047.

20. Hall MH, Campbell DM, Fraser C, Lemon J. Mode of delivery and future fertility. *Br J Obstet Gynaecol* 1989; **96**(11): 1297–1303

21. Murphy DJ, Stirrat GM, Heron J and the ALSPAC Study Team. The relationship between Caesarean section and subfertility in a population-based sample of 14,541 pregnancies. *Hum Reprod* 2002; **17**: 1914–1917.

22. Lydon-Rochelle M, Holt VL, Easterling TR, Martin DP. Risk of uterine rupture during labor among women with a prior Caesarean delivery. *N Engl J Med* 2001; **345**: 54–55.

23. Kadar N, Romero R. Prognosis for future childbearing after mid-cavity instrumental deliveries in primigravidas. *Obstet Gynecol* 1983; **62**: 166–170.

24. Fynes M, Donnelly V, Behan M, O'Connell PR, O'Herlihy C. Effect of second vaginal delivery on anorectal physiology and faecal continence: a prospective study. *Lancet* 1999; **354**: 983–986.

25. Fitzpatrick M, Cassidy M, O'Connell PR, O'Herlihy C. Experience with an obstetric perineal clinic. *Eur J Obstet Gynecol Reprod Biol* 2002; **100**: 199–203.

26. Chiswick ML, James DK. Kielland's forceps: association with neonatal morbidity and mortality. *BMJ* 1979; **1**: 7–9.

27. Okunwobi-Smith Y, Cooke I, MacKenzie IZ. Decision to delivery intervals for assisted vaginal vertex delivery. *Br J Obstet Gynaecol* 2000; **107**: 467–471.

28. Impey L, Greenwood C, MacQuillan K, Reynolds M, Sheil O. Fever in labour and neonatal encephalopathy: a prospective cohort study. *Br J Obstet Gynaecol* 2001; **108**: 594–597.

29. Badawi N, Kurinczuk JJ, Keogh JM *et al*. Intrapartum risk factors for newborn encephalopathy: the Western Australian case-control study. *BMJ* 1998; **317**: 1554–1558.

30. Towner D, Castro MA, Eby-Wilkens E, Gilbert WM. Effect of mode of delivery in nulliparous women on neonatal intracranial injury. *N Engl J Med* 1999; 341: 1709–1714.

Hassan N. Sallam

8

The evidence-based practice of assisted reproduction

In vitro fertilization (IVF) and intracytoplasmic sperm injection (ICSI) are now established methods for the treatment of infertility in a multitude of clinical conditions. However, pregnancy can only be achieved in a fraction of patients undergoing these procedures. In order to improve the results, many modifications have been suggested, but not all of these have been substantiated by randomized controlled trials (RCTs). This chapter will review these modifications in the light of clinical evidence.

STIMULATION PROTOCOLS

The first successful IVF was achieved in a natural non-stimulated cycle.[1] However, it soon became clear that controlled ovarian hyperstimulation resulted in the recruitment of more oocytes and better pregnancy rates (Table 1). Controlled ovarian hyperstimulation was first achieved with clomiphene citrate, but this was later superseded with the use of human menopausal gonadotrophins (HMGs) and urinary FSH preparations.[2] Nevertheless, the results were hampered by the possibility of premature luteinization leading to cancellation of many treatment cycles.

The introduction of GnRH agonists (GnRHa) permitted the down-regulation of the pituitary gland in order to eliminate any premature LH surge and various protocols have been suggested and used successfully.[3,4] In the short protocols of GnRHa administration, the agonist is started on day 1 or 2 of the menstrual cycle. The injection of HMG is commenced a few days after the start of GnRHa, and the agonist is continued until the day of HCG administration. In the ultrashort protocol, the agonist is administered for 2 or 3 days only at the beginning of the cycle in order to take advantage of its flare-

Hassan N. Sallam MB ChB DGO DrChO&G(Alex) FRCOG PhD, Professor in Obstetrics and Gynaecology, University of Alexandria, 22 Victor Emanuel Square, Smouha, Alexandria, Egypt

Table 1 Odds ratios and 95% confidence intervals for the clinical pregnancy rate with various stimulation protocols for patients treated with IVF

Stimulation protocol	Odds ratio (95% CI)
Urinary FSH *versus* HMG stimulation[2]	1.70 (1.11–2.60)
Long *versus* short and ultrashort protocols[3]	1.32 (1.10–1.57)
Long *versus* short protocols[3]	1.27 (1.04–1.56)
Long *versus* ultrashort protocols[3]	1.47 (1.02–2.12)
GnRH agonists *versus* HMG stimulation[4]	1.80 (1.33–2.44)
GnRH antagonists *versus* agonists[5]	0.79 (0.63–0.99)
Recombinant *versus* urinary FSH[6]	1.21 (1.04–1.42)

up effect and the HMG is started afterwards. In the long protocols, HMG administration is delayed until pituitary desensitization has been achieved, usually 2–3 weeks. In these long protocols, GnRHa is started either in the midluteal phase or in the early follicular phase.

More recently, GnRH antagonists were introduced with various claims of success. These compounds do not have a flare-up effect and down-regulation is achieved immediately. Two protocols for GnRH antagonists have been described: the single-dose protocol and the multiple-dose protocol. In the single dose protocol, one single dose of 3 mg is administered in the late follicular phase, while in the multiple-dose protocol, the effect is achieved by daily administration of 0.25 mg of the antagonists, starting on day 5 or 6 of the cycle.[5]

GNRH AGONISTS *VERSUS* HMG

It has now been established that the routine use of GnRHa prior to IVF and gamete intrafallopian transfer (GIFT) increases the clinical pregnancy rate compared to the use of HMG alone. In a meta-analysis of RCTs, Hughes *et al.* found that the clinical pregnancy rate per cycle commenced was significantly improved after GnRHa use for IVF (common odds ratio, 1.80; 95% CI, 1.33–2.44) and GIFT (common odds ratio, 2.37; 95% CI, 1.24–4.51).[4] Cycle cancellation was decreased (common odds ratio, 0.33; 95% CI, 0.25–0.44), whereas spontaneous abortion was similar with and without GnRHa use. However, GnRHa was associated with a slight, but insignificant, increase in the incidence of ovarian hyperstimulation syndrome and multiple pregnancies (common odds ratio, 2.56; 95% CI, 0.95–6.91).

LONG *VERSUS* SHORT PROTOCOLS

Randomized controlled trials have shown that long stimulation protocols are superior to short and ultrashort stimulation protocols in terms of clinical pregnancies. In a Cochrane Review conducted by Daya, the long protocols were compared to the short and ultrashort protocols.[3] The common odds ratio for clinical pregnancy per cycle started was 1.32 (95% CI, 1.10–1.57) in favour of the long GnRHa protocols. When in the long protocol, the GnRHa was commenced in the follicular phase, the respective odds ratios were 1.54 (95% CI, 1.11–2.13) and when the GnRHa was started in luteal phase, the respective odds ratios were 1.21 (95% CI, 0.98–1.51). When the long protocols were compared to the short protocols, the odds ratios were 1.27 (95% CI, 1.04–1.56) in favour of the long protocols. Similarly, when the long protocols were compared to the ultrashort protocols, the odds ratios were 1.47 (95% CI, 1.02–2.12), in favour of the long protocol.

GNRH ANTAGONISTS *VERSUS* AGONISTS

Contrary to expectations, the GnRH antagonist protocols did not improve the clinical pregnancy rates compared to the long stimulation protocols, at least with the regimens studied. In a Cochrane Review conducted by Al-Inany and Aboulghar, five trials fulfilled the inclusion criteria.[5] The reviewers found that, in comparison to the long protocol of GnRHa, the overall odds ratio for the prevention of premature LH surges was 1.76 (95% CI, 0.75–4.16), which is not statistically significant. There were significantly fewer clinical pregnancies in patients treated with GnRH antagonists compared to those treated with the agonists (odds ratio, 0.79; 95% CI, 0.63–0.99). Moreover, there was no statistically significant reduction in incidence of severe ovarian hyperstimulation syndrome, (RR, 0.51; 95% CI, 0.22–1.18) using antagonist regimens as compared to the long GnRHa protocol.

URINARY FSH *VERSUS* HMG

HMG preparations contain FSH and LH in the ratio of 1:1, while urinary FSH preparations contain very small amounts of LH. This suggests that the follicles may be exposed to high levels of LH during their early stages of development when stimulated with HMG compared to the urinary FSH preparations. Many studies have demonstrated that too much LH during the time of follicle development and in the peri-ovulatory phase is associated with reduced rates of fertilization and pregnancy and an increase in the probability of spontaneous abortion.[2]

In a Cochrane Review, Daya compared the use of FSH to HMG in assisted reproduction.[2] He found that the CPR was higher when urinary FSH was used compared to HMG. The overall odds ratio in favour of FSH for cycle start, oocyte retrieval, and embryo transfer were 1.70 (95% CI, 1.11–2.60), 1.68 (95% CI, 1.10–2.56), and 1.69 (95% CI, 1.10–2.59), respectively.

RECOMBINANT FSH *VERSUS* URINARY FSH

The main source of HMG and FSH preparation is the urine of postmenopausal women. New developments in drug manufacturing have resulted in the production of FSH *in vitro* by recombinant DNA technology. These preparations have an extremely high purity and batch-to-batch consistency which make them attractive alternatives to HMG and urinary FSH preparations.

In 2000, Daya and Gunby conducted a Cochrane Review comparing the use of recombinant *versus* urinary FSH preparations in assisted reproduction. They demonstrated a statistically significant increase in clinical pregnancy rate per cycle started with recombinant FSH compared to urinary FSH.[6] This benefit was observed only in standard IVF cycles and not in cycles in which ICSI was used (odds ratio, 1.21; 95% CI, 1.04–1.42). The odds ratio for on-going pregnancy per cycle started was 1.29 (95% CI, 1.08–1.54). There was no significant difference between recombinant and urinary FSH in the rates of spontaneous abortion, multiple pregnancy or OHSS.

NATURAL CYCLES IVF *VERSUS* STIMULATION PROTOCOLS

Despite the fact that the first successful IVF resulted from a natural (non-stimulated) cycle, many subsequent non-randomised studies showed that the clinical pregnancy rate was much higher in stimulated cycles. These results were later confirmed in a RCT comparing the outcome of IVF performed during natural cycles to clomiphene-stimulated cycles.[7] It has also been suggested that performing IVF during natural cycles may improve the outcome in poor responders, endometriosis and in cases of unexplained infertility, but these claims have not been supported by RCTs. However, the real advantages of assisted reproduction performed during natural cycles nowadays are its lower cost and the absence of hyperstimulation. In 2001, Nargund *et al.* performed an economic analysis and calculated that the cost of a natural cycle IVF was approximately 23% of the cost of a stimulated cycle.[8]

PATIENTS WITH POLYCYSTIC OVARIES

In a RCT, MacDougall *et al.* found that patients with ultrasound evidence of polycystic ovaries undergoing assisted reproduction had significantly higher serum oestradiol levels, developed more follicles and produced more oocytes compared to patients with normal looking ovaries.[9] The fertilization rate was significantly reduced in these patients, but the pregnancy rate was not affected. More importantly, they had a significantly higher incidence of ovarian hyperstimulation syndrome. However, there is so far no evidence-based consensus on the best stimulation protocol for this specific group of patients undergoing assisted reproduction in order to diminish the incidence of hyperstimulation.

LABORATORY ISSUES

In order to optimize the results of assisted reproduction, various laboratory modifications have been suggested. These include performing ICSI rather than IVF for all oocytes, even in cases of non-male factor infertility, using co-culturing techniques, assisted hatching techniques, as well as selecting the embryos with the best potential for implantation based on their morphology or by prolonging their culture *in vitro* to the blastocyst stage.

ICSI *VERSUS* IVF IN NON-MALE FACTOR INFERTILITY

In a Cochrane Review, van Rumstke *et al.* found that, in couples with borderline semen, ICSI results in higher fertilization rates per oocyte injected (odds ratio, 3.90; 95% CI, 2.96–5.15) and per oocyte retrieved (odds ratio, 3.79; 95% CI, 2.97-4.85), compared to conventional IVF.[10] They also found that, in couples with normal semen parameters, ICSI results in higher fertilization rates per oocyte injected (odds ratio, 1.42; 95% CI, 1.17–1.72) but not per oocyte retrieved (odds ratio, 0.88; 95% CI, 0.76–1.03) compared to conventional IVF. Consequently, it has been suggested that performing IVF and ICSI on sibling oocytes for patients with non-male factor infertility could improve the outcome of assisted reproduction. A clinical review of four RCTs found that this approach improved the fertilization rate significantly and prevented total fertilization failure in these patients.[11]

CO-CULTURES AND GROUP CULTURE

It has been suggested that culturing human embryos in the presence of other cells could improve the cleavage rate and hence the pregnancy and implantation rates. Various co-culture systems have been used including the Vero cell line, granulosa cells as well as autologous cryopreserved endometrial cells.[12] Many of these RCTs have reported improvement in the cleavage rate, embryo morphology and blastocyst formation rate. However, their clinical value in terms of improving pregnancy rates has not been established. Similarly, it has been suggested that culturing the embryos in groups improves the clinical pregnancy rate but RCTs failed to confirm this observation.[13]

EMBRYO SELECTION

Different methods of embryo selection have been suggested in order to maximize the implantation rate, while diminishing the incidence of multiple pregnancies. Embryos can be selected at the pronuclear stage based on the polarity of the nucleoli inside the two pronuclei. At the 2 or 4 cell stage, embryo selection is based on the size and regularity of the blastomeres and the presence of fragments or on the zona pellucida thickness variation. Scoring of the blastocyst stage embryo has also been described.[14] However, the clinical value of embryo selection based on these scoring systems has not been established by RCTs. More recently, Gianaroli *et al.* performed pre-implantation diagnosis on the embryos by fluorescence *in situ* hybridization (FISH) to exclude embryos with abnormal chromosomes. In this small RCT, the implantation rate increased significantly to 28% compared to 11.9% in the control group.[15] However, this interesting work has not been confirmed by larger RCTs.

ASSISTED HATCHING AND FRAGMENT REMOVAL

It has been suggested that assisted hatching can improve the implantation capacity of the embryos. Assisted hatching can be performed mechanically, chemically (using a microjet of acid Tyrode) or using the Erbium-YAG laser. The technique is usually reserved for older patients (> 40 years), patients with thick or abnormal zona pellucida, and patients with repeated implantation failures. The results of RCTs have been controversial and there is a need for conducting a large, multicentre, randomized study to establish the real value of the technique.[16] Removing cytoplasmic fragments from fragmented embryos has also been claimed to improve clinical pregnancy and implantation rates, but this has not been substantiated by RCTs.[17]

DAY 3 TRANSFER AND BLASTOCYST CULTURE

Prolonged culture of the embryos has been suggested as a method for selecting the embryos with the best potential for survival and hence improving the implantation rates. However, RCTs did not find significant changes in clinical pregnancy or implantation rates when the embryos were replaced on day 3 compared to day 2 after oocyte retrieval.[18] Similarly, RCTs comparing the transfer of the embryos at the blastocyst stage to day 2 or 3 transfer showed no significant improvement in pregnancy rates.[19] However, the real advantage of blastocyst stage transfer is the reduction of multiple pregnancies, as fewer embryos are replaced.[19]

IN VITRO MATURATION

In vitro maturation (IVM) of human oocytes was suggested in order to achieve fertilization of immature oocytes occasionally retrieved during stimulated cycles, oocytes retrieved from PCO patients in natural as well as stimulated cycles, and also after freezing-thawing of immature oocytes. The technique can lead to normal fertilization, embryo development, pregnancies and the delivery of healthy children. However, the overall efficiency is still very low, indicating that embryo viability is compromised. For the majority of patients in need of assisted reproduction, the technique offers no advantages in terms of clinical pregnancy and implantation rates.[20]

OTHER LABORATORY ISSUES

It has been suggested that a high oxygen concentration is detrimental to embryo culture *in vitro*, but RCTs failed to confirm this observation. On the contrary, RCTs have shown that culturing human embryos in antibiotic-free media improves the cleavage rates and that prolonged exposure of the oocytes to the sperm during IVF was associated with lower fertilization rates.[21]

EMBRYO TRANSFER

Embryo transfer is the least successful step in assisted reproduction and 85% of the embryos replaced in the uterine cavity fail to implant. Various techniques have been suggested in order to optimize this apparently simple step, including performing a trial embryo transfer prior to the actual procedure, performing the transfer under ultrasound guidance, using soft catheters rather than the rigid ones, and asking the patients to rest in bed following the transfer.

DUMMY (TRIAL) EMBRYO TRANSFERS

It has been suggested that performing a trial embryo transfer in the cycle preceding the actual procedure could improve the outcome of assisted reproduction and this hypothesis has been confirmed by a RCT. In 1990, Mansour *et al.* conducted this trial and found that the clinical pregnancy and implantation rates increased significantly in those patients who had a trial embryo transfer compared to those who did not (22.8% *versus* 13.1%, $P < 0.05$ and 7.2% *versus* 4.2%, $P < 0.05$, respectively).[22]

ULTRASOUND-GUIDED EMBRYO TRANSFER

Many studies have reported that ultrasound-guided embryo transfer is associated with an increase in the clinical pregnancy and implantation rates. We have recently conducted a meta-analysis of RCTs and found that ultrasound-guided embryo transfer increased the clinical pregnancy rate significantly (odds ratio, 1.198; 95% CI, 1.018–1.410) as well as the implantation rate (odds ratio, 1.327; 95% CI, 1 168–1.507) and the on-going pregnancy rate (odds ratio, 1.456; 95% CI, 1136–1866).[23]

Ultrasound-guided embryo transfer is mainly used to confirm that the embryos are properly deposited in the uterine fundus and to follow the embryo-associated air bubble afterwards. We have also suggested that ultrasound can be used to measure the uterocervical angle (Fig. 1) and mould the embryo transfer catheter according to this angle. In a prospective controlled trial, we have found that this technique increased the clinical pregnancy (odds ratio, 1.57; 95% CI, 1.08–2.27) and implantation rates (odds ratio, 1.47; 95% CI, 1.10–1.96) significantly compared to the 'clinical touch method'.[24] The incidences of difficult transfers (odds ratio, 0.25; 95% CI, 0.16–0.40) and blood (odds ratio, 0.71; 95% CI, 0.50–0.99) during transfers were also significantly reduced.

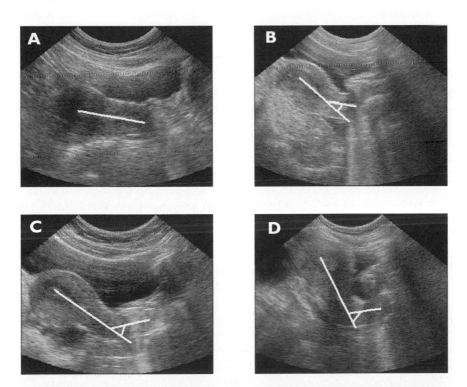

Fig. 1 Measuring the uterocervical angle prior to embryo transfer. (A) No angle; (B) small angle (< 30°); (C) moderate angle (30–60°); (D) large angle (> 60°). Reproduced with the kind permission of the Editor of *Human Reproduction*.

SOFT CATHETERS *VERSUS* RIGID CATHETERS

Different types of embryo transfer catheters have been used in assisted reproduction with various claims of success. In particular, it has been suggested that soft catheters do not indent the uterine fundus and result in higher clinical pregnancy rates.[25] However, these claims have not yet been substantiated by other RCTs. Larger RCTs are, therefore, necessary to determine the superiority or otherwise of any particular embryo transfer catheter.

SITE OF EMBRYO DEPOSITION

It has been suggested that depositing the embryos too near to the uterine fundus could risk injuring the endometrium and diminish the outcome of assisted reproduction and this hypothesis has recently been supported by a RCT. In this study, Coroleu *et al.* reported a significantly higher implantation rate when the embryos were deposited 2 cm below the uterine fundus compared to when deposited 1 cm below the fundus ($P < 0.05$).[26]

BED REST AFTER EMBRYO TRANSFER

Prolonged bed rest after embryo transfer does not improve the outcome of assisted reproduction. In 1997, Botta *et al.* conducted a RCT of 182 patients undergoing embryo transfer and found no statistically significant difference in clinical pregnancy rates between patients who rested in bed for 24 h after transfer compared to those who rested for 20 min only.[27]

OTHER FACTORS AFFECTING EMBRYO TRANSFER

It has also been suggested that cervical infection is detrimental to assisted reproduction. In an observational study, Egbase *et al.* cultured the tip of the embryo transfer catheter and found that the clinical pregnancy rate was significantly lower for patients with positive cultures compared to those with negative cultures.[28] When antibiotics were routinely administered to patients with positive cultures, the clinical pregnancy and implantation rates improved significantly (from 17.8% to 41.3%, $P < 0.01$ and from 9.3% to 21.6%, $P < 0.001$, respectively). However, the value of routine administration of antibiotics has not been tested in a RCT.

On the contrary, RCTs have shown that waiting for 30 s before withdrawing the embryo transfer catheter and vigorous flushing of the cervical canal with culture medium before embryo transfer do not improve the clinical pregnancy rate.[29]

IMPLANTATION AND ENDOMETRIAL RECEPTIVITY

Medawar defined implantation as an immunological paradox whereby the semi-allograft human conceptus, immunologically foreign to the mother, evades immune rejection to penetrate and imbed in the semi-foreign endometrium. This fact is very much highlighted during assisted reproduction and various attempts have been made to improve endometrial receptivity in order to increase the clinical pregnancy and implantation rates. These include

Table 2 Odds ratio and 95% confidence intervals for the clinical pregnancy rate with various factors affecting implantation for patients treated with IVF

Stimulation protocol	Odds ratio (95% CI)
HCG *versus* no HCG in GnRH agonist protocols[30]	4.2 (1.9–9.1)
Progesterone *versus* no progesterone in all protocols[30]	1.2 (1.0–1.7)
HCG *versus* progesterone in GnRH agonist protocols[30]	2.0 (1.1–3.9)
Hydrosalpinx *versus* no hydrosalpinx in IVF patients[32]	0.64 (0.56–0.74)
Removal of hydrosalpinx *versus* no removal[34]	1.75 (1.07–2.86)
Endometriosis *versus* tubal factor infertility[35]	0.81 (0.72–0.91)
Stages III and IV *versus* stages I and II endometriosis[35]	0.60 (0.42–0.87)

various regimens of luteal support, the use of corticosteroids, the removal of hydrosalpinges, diminishing uterine contractions as well as enhancing the endometrial blood flow (Table 2).

PROGESTERONE *VERSUS* HCG SUPPLEMENTATION

It has been suggested that the use of GnRHa down-regulation protocols could result in luteal phase insufficiency during assisted reproduction. In order to counteract this effect, luteal phase support has been used both by progesterone supplementation and/or HCG administration. In a meta-analysis of RCTs, Soliman *et al.* found that HCG administration improved the clinical pregnancy rate significantly in patients receiving GnRHa stimulation protocols (common odds ratio, 4.2; 95% CI, 1.9–9.1). However, this effect could not be evaluated in patients receiving other stimulation protocols due to the heterogeneity of the studies. On the contrary, they found that progesterone supplementation increased the clinical pregnancy rate significantly with all stimulation protocols (common odds ratio, 1.2; 95% CI, 1.0–1.7). When both luteal support methods were compared, HCG administration was superior to progesterone supplementation when GnRHa was used (common odds ratio, 2.0; 95% CI, 1.1–3.9), but not with other stimulation regimens.[30]

CORTICOSTEROIDS

Clinical studies have suggested that the administration of corticosteroids during IVF therapy might improve the clinical pregnancy rate.[31] However, different corticosteroid preparations were used in these studies and further RCTs using comparable preparations are necessary in order to confirm or refute these interesting observations.

REMOVAL OF HYDROSALPINGES

Various studies have shown that the presence of a hydrosalpinx has a detrimental effect on the outcome of assisted reproduction, apparently because the tubal fluid accumulates inside the uterine cavity. In 1999, Camus *et al.* conducted a meta-analysis of published studies and showed that the clinical pregnancy rate was significantly lower in patients with hydrosalpinges undergoing assisted reproductive measures compared to those with no hydrosalpinges (odds ratio, 0.64; 95% CI, 0.56–0.74). The implantation rate was also diminished (odds ratio, 0.63; 95% CI, 0.55–0.72) as was the delivery rate (odds ratio, 0.58; 95% CI, 0.49–0.69). Pregnancy loss was also significantly higher in patients with hydrosalpinges (odds ratio, 1.78; 95% CI, 1.31–2.48).[32]

Consequently, the removal of hydrosalpinges prior to assisted reproduction has been suggested as a measure to improve the outcome. A RCT conducted by Strandell *et al.* showed that the removal of the fallopian tubes in patients with bilateral hydrosalpinges increased their implantation, clinical pregnancy and delivery rates significantly ($P < 0.05$ in all cases).[33] The removal of a unilateral hydrosalpinx also increased the implantation and pregnancy rates, but this did not reach statistical significance, probably because the study lacked enough power.

More recently, a Cochrane Review conducted by Johnson *et al.* showed that laparoscopic salpingectomy significant increased the clinical pregnancy rate (odds ratio, 1.75; 95% CI, 1.07–2.86) as well as the live birth rate (odds ratio, 2.13; (95% CI, 1.24–3.65).[34] The implantation rate was also increased and the ectopic pregnancy and miscarriage rates were diminished, but these changes did not reach statistical significance.

ENDOMETRIOSIS AND ASSISTED REPRODUCTION

A recent meta-analysis has shown that patients with endometriosis-associated infertility undergoing assisted reproduction have significantly lower pregnancy rates compared to patients with tubal factor infertility (odds ratio, 0.81; 95% CI, 0.72–0.91).[35] Moreover, patients with stages III and IV endometriosis have a lower pregnancy rate compared to those with stages I and II (odds ratio, 0.60; 95% CI, 0.42–0.87). However, no evidence-based consensus has so far been reached on the best strategy to improve pregnancy rates in those patients.

FIBROMYOMATA AND ASSISTED REPRODUCTION

The effect of fibromyomata on the results of assisted reproduction is still a matter of controversy. While some RCTs have shown that the clinical pregnancy rates are diminished in these patients, other studies have not confirmed this effect particularly when the fibromyoma is not affecting the uterine cavity.[36] There is, therefore, a need for large RCTs in order to resolve the issue and determine whether treatment of the fibromyomata prior to assisted reproduction is necessary.

OTHER FACTORS AFFECTING IMPLANTATION

Uterine contractions during embryo transfer have been blamed for diminishing the outcome of assisted reproduction. In an observational study, Fanchin *et al.* recorded uterine contraction during embryo transfer and found that fewer uterine contractions were associated with a higher clinical pregnancy rate. They also found that plasma progesterone concentrations and the frequency of uterine contractions were negatively correlated (r, –0.34; $P < 0.001$).[37] However, no RCT has so far been published on the use of uterine relaxants during embryo transfer.

Sexual intercourse around the time of embryo transfer has also been suggested as a cause of low implantation rates after assisted reproduction. However, when a RCT was conducted by Tremellen *et al.*, the clinical pregnancy rate was not affected by sexual intercourse and, contrary to expectations, the implantation rate was significantly increased for patients who had sexual intercourse around the time of embryo transfer.[38]

Endometrial echogenicity and vascularity were also studied for patients undergoing assisted reproduction. In a prospective study of 405 patients, Coulam *et al.* found that ultrasonic measurements of pulsatility index, resistance index, and the echogenic pattern were useful in predicting implantation after assisted reproduction, but these results were not confirmed in subsequent studies.[39] In an attempt to increase endometrial vascularity, Sher and Fisch used sildenafil (Viagra) in 4 patients with previously failed IVF attempts and 3 of them conceived.[40] However, to date, no RCTs have been published to confirm this interesting observation. On the contrary, a RCT showed that the administration of low-dose aspirin did not improve implantation and pregnancy rates for patients undergoing ICSI.[41]

CONCLUSIONS

The multifaceted nature of assisted reproduction requires a meticulous evidence-based approach to the various steps involved in this treatment modality. With the ever-increasing numbers of patients in need of assisted reproduction, the clinical pregnancy rate can only be improved by relying on properly conducted RCTs.

Key points for clinical practice

- GnRHa down-regulation protocols are associated with higher clinical pregnancy rates compared to HMG-only protocols and the long protocols are superior to the short ones.

- GnRH antagonists protocols are not better than GnRHa protocols.

- Urinary FSH is better than HMG and recombinant FSH is better that urinary FSH.

- Natural cycle IVF is associated with lower pregnancy rates compared to controlled ovarian stimulation protocols, but is cheaper and does not produce hyperstimulation.

- Performing IVF and ICSI on sibling oocytes for patients with non-male factor infertility improves the fertilization rate and prevents total fertilization failure.

- For the majority of patients, RCTs have not so far shown any clinical advantage in using co-cultures, group culture, *in vitro* maturation or assisted hatching. Embryo selection methods and blastocyst culture do not improve pregnancy rates but diminish the incidence of multiple pregnancies. (continued on next page)

Key points for clinical practice (continued)

- RCTs have shown that ultrasound-guided embryo transfer, a trial transfer prior to the actual procedure and depositing the embryos 2 cm below the uterine fundus are associated with higher pregnancy rates. Bed rest and sexual intercourse do not affect the results.

- The value of using soft catheters, vigorous flushing of the cervical canal and the routine use of antibiotics has not been established.

- RCTs have established that the removal of any hydrosalpinx before assisted reproduction improves the clinical pregnancy rates. Endometriosis diminishes the clinical pregnancy rate and patients with polycystic ovaries have normal pregnancy rates but are liable to hyperstimulation.

- Progesterone supplementation increases the clinical pregnancy rates in all protocols, HCG increases the pregnancy rates in GnRHa protocols and HCG is superior to progesterone in GnRHa protocols. The value of using corticosteroids, uterine muscle relaxants, sildenafil and aspirin has not been established.

References

1. Steptoe PC, Edwards RG. Birth after the re-implantation of a human embryo. *Lancet* 1978; **2**: 366.
2. Daya S. Follicle-stimulating hormone and human menopausal gonadotropin for ovarian stimulation in assisted reproduction cycles. In: Daya S. (ed) *Gonadotrophin-releasing hormone agonist protocols for pituitary desensitization in in vitro fertilization and gamete intrafallopian transfer cycles* (Cochrane Review). In: Oxford: The Cochrane Library, Issue 1, 2002.
3. Daya S. *Gonadotrophin-releasing hormone agonist protocols for pituitary desensitization in in vitro fertilization and gamete intrafallopian transfer cycles* (Cochrane Review). Oxford: The Cochrane Library, Issue 1, 2002.
4. Hughes EG, Fedorkow DM, Daya S *et al*. The routine use of gonadotropin-releasing hormone agonists prior to *in vitro* fertilization and gamete intrafallopian transfer: a meta-analysis of randomized controlled trials. *Fertil Steril* 1992; **58**: 888–896.
5. Al-Inany H, Aboulghar M. Gonadotrophin-releasing hormone antagonists for assisted conception. In: Daya S. (ed) *Gonadotrophin-releasing hormone agonist protocols for pituitary desensitization in in vitro fertilization and gamete intrafallopian transfer cycles* (Cochrane Review). In: Oxford: The Cochrane Library, Issue 1, 2002.
6. Daya S, Gunby J. Recombinant versus urinary follicle stimulating hormone for ovarian stimulation in assisted reproduction cycles. In: Daya S. (ed) *Gonadotrophin-releasing hormone agonist protocols for pituitary desensitization in in vitro fertilization and gamete intrafallopian transfer cycles* (Cochrane Review). In: Oxford: The Cochrane Library, Issue 1, 2002.
7. MacDougall MJ, Tan SL, Hall V et al. Comparison of natural with clomiphene citrate-stimulated cycles in in vitro fertilization: a prospective, randomized trial. *Fertil Steril* 1994; **61**: 1052–1057.
8. Nargund G, Waterstone J, Bland J, et al. Cumulative conception and live birth rates in natural (unstimulated) IVF cycles. *Hum Reprod* 2001; **16**: 259–262.
9. MacDougall MJ, Tan SL, Balen A, Jacobs HS. A controlled study on comparing patients with and without polycystic ovaries undergoing in vitro fertilization. *Hum Reprod* 1993; **8**: 233–237.

10. van Rumste MME, Evers JLH, Farquhar CM, Blake DA. Intra-cytoplasmic sperm injection versus partial zona dissection, subzonal insemination and conventional techniques for oocyte insemination during in vitro fertilisation. In: Daya S. (ed) *Gonadotrophin-releasing hormone agonist protocols for pituitary desensitization in in vitro fertilization and gamete intrafallopian transfer cycles* (Cochrane Review). In: Oxford: The Cochrane Library, Issue 1, 2002.

11. Khamsi F, Yavas Y, Roberge S et al. The status of controlled prospective clinical trials for efficacy of intracytoplasmic sperm injection in in vitro fertilization for non-male factor infertility. *J Assist Reprod Genet* 2000; **17**: 504–507.

12. Veiga A, Torello MJ, Menezo Y et al. Use of co-culture of human embryos on Vero cells to improve clinical implantation rate. *Hum Reprod* 1999; **14 (Suppl 2)**: 112–120.

13. Spyropoulou I, Karamalegos C, Bolton VN. A prospective randomized study comparing the outcome of in vitro fertilization and embryo transfer following culture of human embryos individually or in groups before embryo transfer on day 2. *Hum Reprod* 1999; **14**: 76–79.

14. Gardner DK, Lane M, Stevens J, Schlenker T, Schoolcraft WB. Blastocyst score affects implantation and pregnancy outcome: towards a single blastocyst transfer. *Fertil Steril* 2000; **73**: 1155–1158.

15. Gianaroli L, Magli MC, Ferraretti AP et al. Pre-implantation genetic diagnosis increases the implantation rate in human in vitro fertilization by avoiding the transfer of chromosomally abnormal embryos. *Fertil Steril* 1997; **68**: 1128–1131.

16. Tucker MJ, Morton PC, Wright G et al. Enhancement of outcome from intracytoplasmic sperm injection: does co-culture or assisted hatching improve implantation rates? *Hum Reprod* 1996; **11**: 2434–1437.

17. Alikani M, Cohen J, Tomkin G et al. Human embryo fragmentation in vitro and its implications for pregnancy and implantation. *Fertil Steril* 1999; **71**: 836–842.

18. Laverge H, De Sutter P, Van der Elst J, Dhont M. A prospective, randomized study comparing day 2 and day 3 embryo transfer in human IVF. *Hum Reprod* 2001; **16**: 476–480.

19. Plachot M, Belaisch-Allart J, Mayenga JM *et al.* Blastocyst stage transfer: the real benefits compared with early embryo transfer. *Hum Reprod* 2000; **15 (Suppl 6)**: 24–30.

20. Plachot M. *In vitro* maturation of human oocytes. *Contracept Fertil Sex* 1999; **27**: 434–439.

21. Dirnfeld M, Bider D, Koifman M, Calderon I, Abramovici H. Shortened exposure of oocytes to spermatozoa improves *in vitro* fertilization outcome: a prospective, randomized, controlled study. *Hum Reprod* 1999; **14**: 2562–2564.

22. Mansour RT, Aboulghar MA, Serour GI, Amin YM. Dummy embryo transfer using methylene blue dye. *Hum Reprod* 1994; **9**: 1257–1259.

23. Sallam HN, Saad-el-Din S. Performing embryo transfer under ultrsound guidance – a meta-analysis of randomized trials. *Fertil Steril* 2002; **78**(Suppl): 46

24. Sallam HN, Agameya AF, Rahman AF, Ezzeldin F, Sallam AN. Ultrasound measurement of the uterocervical angle before embryo transfer: a prospective controlled study. *Hum Reprod* 2002; **17**: 1767–1772.

25. van Weering HG, Schats R, McDonnell J *et al.* The impact of the embryo transfer catheter on the pregnancy rate in IVF. *Hum Reprod* 2002; **17**: 666–670.

26. Coroleu B, Barri PN, Carreras O *et al.* The influence of the depth of embryo replacement into the uterine cavity on implantation rates after IVF: a controlled, ultrasound-guided study. *Hum Reprod* 2002; **17**: 341–346.

27. Botta G, Grudzinskas G. Is a prolonged bed rest following embryo transfer useful? *Hum Reprod* 1997; **12**: 2489–2492.

28. Egbase PE, Udo EE, Al-Sharhan M, Grudzinskas JG. Prophylactic antibiotics and endocervical microbial inoculation of the endometrium at embryo transfer. *Lancet* 1999; **354**: 651–652.

29. Sallam HN, Farrag F, Ezzeldin A, Agameya A, Sallam AN. The importance of flushing the cervical canal with culture medium prior to embryo transfer. *Fertil Steril* 2000; **74**(Suppl 1): 64–65.

30. Soliman S, Daya S, Collins J, Hughes EG. The role of luteal phase support in infertility treatment: a meta-analysis of randomized trials. *Fertil Steril* 1994; **61**: 1068–1076.

31. Bider D, Amoday I, Tur-Kaspa I, Livshits A, Dor J. The addition of a glucocorticoid to the protocol of programmed oocyte retrieval for *in vitro* fertilization – a randomized study. *Hum Reprod* 1996; **11**: 1606–1608.

32. Camus E, Poncelet C, Goffinet F *et al*. Pregnancy rates after *in vitro* fertilization in cases of tubal infertility with and without hydrosalpinx: a meta-analysis of published comparative studies. *Hum Reprod* 1999; **14**: 1243–1249.

33. Strandell A, Lindhard A, Waldenstrom U *et al*. Hydrosalpinx and IVF outcome: a prospective, randomized multicentre trial in Scandinavia on salpingectomy prior to IVF. *Hum Reprod* 1999; **14**: 2762–2769.

34. Johnson NP, Mak W, Sowter MC. Surgical treatment for tubal disease in women due to undergo *in vitro* fertilisation. In: Daya S. (ed) *Gonadotrophin-releasing hormone agonist protocols for pituitary desensitization in in vitro fertilization and gamete intrafallopian transfer cycles* (Cochrane Review). In: Oxford: The Cochrane Library, Issue 1, 2002.

35. Barnhart K, Dunsmoor-Su R, Coutifaris C. Effect of endometriosis on *in vitro* fertilization. *Fertil Steril* 2002; **77**: 1148–1155.

36. Hart R, Khalaf Y, Yeong CT *et al*. A prospective controlled study of the effect of intramural uterine fibroids on the outcome of assisted conception. *Hum Reprod* 2001; **16**: 2411–2417.

37. Fanchin R, Righini C, Olivennes F *et al*. Uterine contractions at the time of embryo transfer alter pregnancy rates after *in vitro* fertilization. *Hum Reprod* 1998; **13**: 1968–1974.

38. Tremellen KP, Valbuena D, Landeras J *et al*. The effect of intercourse on pregnancy rates during assisted human reproduction. *Hum Reprod* 2000; **15**: 2653–2658.

39. Coulam CB, Bustillo M, Soenksen DM, Britten S. Ultrasonographic predictors of implantation after assisted reproduction. *Fertil Steril* 1994; **62**: 1004–1010.

40. Sher G, Fisch JD. Vaginal sildenafil (Viagra): a preliminary report of a novel method to improve uterine artery blood flow and endometrial development in patients undergoing IVF. *Hum Reprod* 2000; **15**: 806–809.

41. Urman B, Mercan R, Alatas C *et al*. Low-dose aspirin does not increase implantation rates in patients undergoing intracytoplasmic sperm injection: a prospective randomized study. *J Assist Reprod Genet* 2000; **17**: 586–590.

Rezan A. Kadir Demetrious L. Economides

9

Menorrhagia and bleeding disorders

Menorrhagia is a significant healthcare problem and has major socio-economic costs. About 5% of women aged 30–49 years consult their general practitioner with this problem which also accounts for 12% of all gynaecology referrals. Menorrhagia has been attributed to a number of local or systemic disorders, but in more than half the women, no organic pathology is found. Heavy menstruation is well recognized in women with bleeding disorders. However, bleeding disorders are usually presumed to be a rare cause of menorrhagia especially in adults. Recently, research and clinical awareness have increased in this area. Identifying bleeding problems in women with menorrhagia and close collaboration between gynaecologists and haematologists in the management of these women is the way forward to improve quality-of-life and avoid unnecessary surgical interventions.

HAEMOSTASIS DURING MENSTRUATION

Haemostasis in the menstruating uterus is the result of a fine balance between platelet aggregation, fibrin formation, vasoconstriction, and tissue regeneration on the one hand, and prostaglandin-induced platelet inhibition, vasodilatation, and fibrinolysis on the other. Haemostasis in the endometrium is characterised by relative scarcity of haemostatic plugs and by the complete intravascular location of these plugs. Numerous thrombi are present in the endometrium during the first 20 h of menstruation, but thereafter most of the functional layer is shed and no more thrombi are seen.[1] Haemostatic plug formation plays an important role in uterine haemostasis during first 2–3 days of menstruation and menstrual loss is increased in patients with primary haemostatic disorders (*e.g.*

Rezan A. Kadir MRCOG FRCS MD, Consultant Obstetrician and Gynaecologist, The Royal Free Hospital School of Medicine, Pond Street, London NW3 2QG, UK (for correspondence)

Demetrious L. Economides FRCOG MD, Consultant Obstetrician and Gynaecologist, The Royal Free Hospital School of Medicine, Pond Street, London NW3 2QG, UK von Willebrand's disease and thrombocytopenia). However, these women bleed heavily throughout menstruation[2] not only for the first 20 h. A possible explanation is that thrombus formation itself promotes tissue shedding. Diminished plug formation could then lead to prolonged endometrial shedding and, because shedding is incomplete, further haemostatic plugs are required for shedding to arrest.[1] Therefore, any disorders of blood coagulation especially those of primary haemostasis (*e.g.* disorders of blood vessels, platelet abnormalities, and von Willebrand's disease) may result in prolonged and excessive menstrual bleeding. In fact, the first patient described with von Willebrand's disease by Erik von Willebrand in 1926 died of uncontrollable menstrual bleeding at the age of 13 years.[3]

Activation of the coagulation cascade (secondary haemostasis) results in the stabilisation of the primary haemostatic plug by fibrin formation from fibrinogen by action of thrombin. Thrombin is formed from prothrombin through the activation of several coagulation factors in the coagulation cascade. Therefore, deficiencies of any of the coagulation factors in the cascade may also be associated with menorrhagia.

MENSTRUAL PROBLEMS IN WOMEN WITH BLEEDING DISORDERS

MENORRHAGIA

We assessed menstrual loss using the pictorial blood assessment chart[4] (Fig. 1) and gynaecological problems in 116 patients with inherited bleeding disorders (von Willebrand's disease, mainly type 1 [*n* = 66], carriers of haemophilia [*n* = 30] and FXI deficiency [*n* = 20]). The incidence of menorrhagia as defined by score of more than 100, was 67% compared to 29% in the age-matched control group. These women also had prolonged menstruation and 25% of them bled for more than 8 days compared to only 4% in the control group.[2] Table 1 shows menstrual scores in women with bleeding disorders. In the same study, we also demonstrated a strong relationship between menstrual blood loss and duration of menstruation indicating that these women bleed heavily throughout their

Table 1 Menstrual scores in women with inherited bleeding disorders and in controls

	Median score	Range	Women with score > 100
Carriers of haemophilia A (*n* = 14)	111	50–482	8 (57.1%)
Carriers of haemophilia B (*n* = 7)	115	53–200	4 (57.1%)
von Willebrand's disease (*n* = 57)	139	55–456	42 (73.7%)
FXI deficiency (*n* = 17)	108	38–424	10 (58.8%)
Total (*n* = 95)	122	38–482	64 (67.4%)*
Control (*n* = 69)	73	9–310	20 (29.0%)*

n, number of women completed PBAC; *statistically significant difference (*P* = 0.001).

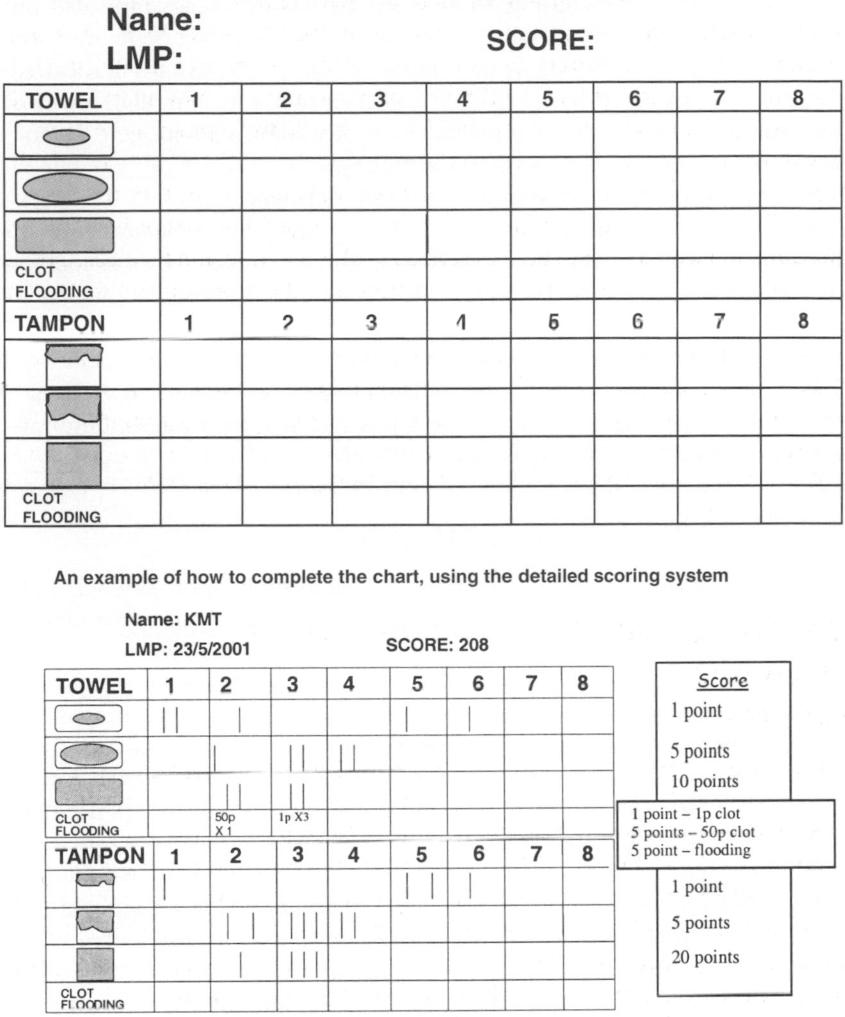

Name:

LMP:

SCORE:

TOWEL	1	2	3	4	5	6	7	8
⬭								
⬭								
▬								
CLOT FLOODING								
TAMPON	1	2	3	4	5	6	7	8
CLOT FLOODING								

An example of how to complete the chart, using the detailed scoring system

Name: KMT

LMP: 23/5/2001   SCORE: 208

TOWEL	1	2	3	4	5	6	7	8		Score
⬭	II	I			I	I				1 point
⬭		I	II	II						5 points
▬		III	II							10 points
CLOT FLOODING		50p X1	1p X3							1 point – 1p clot 5 points – 50p clot 5 point – flooding
TAMPON	1	2	3	4	5	6	7	8		
	I				I I	I				1 point
		I I	III	II						5 points
			I	III						20 points
CLOT FLOODING										

Fig. 1 Pictorial blood assessment chart and scoring system for assessment of menstrual blood loss.

menstruation. This is in contrast to women with menorrhagia without bleeding disorders, where 90% of the total menstrual loss is in the first 3 days.[5]

The high prevalence of menorrhagia among women with von Willebrand's disease has been reported in several studies. In a survey of 99 patients with type 1 von Willebrand's disease from four haemophilia centres in the US, 78% reported their periods to be heavy, 71% of whom required medical attention and 15% who required hysterectomy.[6] In a study by Ragni et al.,[7] 93% of the 38 women with von Willebrand's disease suffered from heavy menstruation. Menorrhagia was also the commonest initial bleeding symptom leading to the diagnosis of the disease in 53% of them and in all this started from menarche.

In carriers of haemophilia, subjective menorrhagia has also been reported[8] although in the study by Mauser Bunschoten et al.[9] there was no significant difference in the percentage of carriers who considered their menstrual loss to be greater than other women compared to a reference group. Women affected with FXI deficiency, including those with partial deficiency, are also more likely to have menorrhagia than their unaffected relatives.[10] In this study, 19/46 (41%) of FXI-deficient women reported symptoms usually indicative of menorrhagia compared with 6/33 (18%) of their non-deficient relatives. Heavy menstruation has also been reported in prothrombin, fibrinogen, Factor V, Factor VII, Factor X and Factor XIII deficiency.

Menorrhagia is also a major cause for iron-deficiency anaemia. This type of anaemia was reported in 64% of 81 menstruating type 1 von Willebrand's disease patients compared to 34% in a menstruating control group.[6] Hysterectomy rate amongst these women is also high – 14% among 431 patients studied by four groups of investigators.[2,6,7,11] Hysterectomy is usually done at a young age. The mean age of hysterectomy in our centre was 38 years and, in the majority, the hysterectomy was performed prior to diagnosis of von Willebrand's disease. In women with von Willebrand's disease types 2 and 3, the hysterectomy rate is higher and reported at 23% by Foster in 1995.[12]

DYSMENORRHEA AND MID-CYCLE PAIN

Moderate-to-severe dysmenorrhea has been reported in approximately half of 180 patients from our centre and upstate New York.[6,13] Non-steroidal anti-inflammatory drugs are used successfully for dysmenorrhea and may also reduce menstrual blood loss in women with menorrhagia. In women with bleeding disorders, especially those with severe deficiency, they may increase menstrual blood loss and cause other bleeding complications due to their anti-platelet effect. Therefore, their use in these women is inappropriate. Cyclo-oxygenase-2 inhibitors could be more appropriate, but their role in dysmenorrhea has not been studied.

Mid-cycle pain (Mittleschmerz syndrome), as severe as patients' menstrual pain, was reported in 49% of type 1 von Willebrand's disease women in the upstate New York study.[6] This pain probably arises from ovulation with subsequent haemorrhage into the corpus luteum or peritoneal irritation due to bleeding from edges of a recently formed corpus luteum. An acute abdomen due to haemoperitoneum and extension of bleeding into the broad ligament with spontaneous rupture of corpus luteum has been reported in patients with bleeding disorders.[14,15] This complication should be considered, especially those with severe deficiency such as type 3 von Willebrand's disease, before embarking on any surgical intervention. Conservative management with factor replacement can avoid surgery.[15]

QUALITY-OF-LIFE

Menorrhagia can be a debilitating social problem for women and have a major influence on women's life-style and employment. Excessive menstrual loss results in more than 300,000 sick days per year in all women of reproductive ages in Sweden.[16] Women's estimates of the expense of menstruation, is reported to be £6 and £8 per period in those with normal or excessive menstruation, respectively.[16]

We studied quality-of-life during menstruation in 99 women with inherited bleeding disorders and 69 control using Modified Short Form 36.[13] Women with inherited bleeding disorders had a significantly worse quality-of-life during menstruation compared to the control group and quality-of-life was the worst among patients with von Willebrand's disease especially those who passed clots, suffered flooding, and had prolonged menstruation. Between 39–46% of these patients lose time from work.[6,13] They also accomplished less at work and experienced difficulties performing their work. A study from Frankfurt found a strong relationship between gynaecological history and psychological problems in 181 women with von Willebrand's disease and 28% of the patients met the criteria for anxiety disorders.[11]

Therefore, von Willebrand's disease is clinically a 'disease of women' as described in 1926 by Eric von Willebrand[3] in his first publication and even mild forms of the disease can be associated with significant gynaecological morbidity.

BLEEDING DISORDERS AS AN UNDERLYING CAUSE FOR MENORRHAGIA

While the prevalence of bleeding disorders in older women with menorrhagia seems to be under-estimated, acute adolescent menorrhagia requiring urgent medical intervention has long been recognised to be associated with bleeding disorders. A primary coagulation disorder was found in almost 20% of 59 adolescents with menorrhagia[17] and screening for von Willebrand's disease and platelet disorders has been recommended in these patients. Recent studies shown in Table 2 have reported the prevalence of bleeding disorders, mainly von Willebrand's disease, in older women with menorrhagia.[18–21] The prevalence of von Willebrand's disease was 10.9% (range, 7–20%) in 339 women compared to a prevalence of 1.3% in the general population.[22] All these studies looked at women with menorrhagia presenting to a gynaecologist.

Table 2 Prevalence studies of von Willebrand's disease in women presenting to gynaecologists with menorrhagia

Author	Number in study	Prevalence of vWD	Comments
Edlund et al.[16]	30	20%	vWF not adjusted for ABO blood type MBL – alkaline haematin method
Kadir et al.[19]	150	13%	vWF not adjusted for ABO blood type MBL – PBAC
Dilley et al.[19]	121	7% in all, 16% in Caucasians	vWF adjusted for ABO blood type MBL – subjective Medical record diagnosis of menorrhagia
Woo et al.[21]	38	13%	vWF not adjusted for ABO blood type MBL – alkaline haematin method
Total	339	10.9%	

vWF, von Willebrand factor; MBL, menstrual blood loss assessment; Prevalence, prevalence of von Willebrand's disease.

These may not represent all women with menorrhagia as general practitioners do not refer all patients to hospital. In addition, these studies have different criteria for diagnosis, which will be discussed later.

These studies raise the important question about testing for von Willebrand's disease or inherited bleeding disorder as part of the routine investigation in menorrhagia. The Royal College of Obstetricians and Gynaecologists (RCOG) guidelines for the management of menorrhagia published in 1999[23] recommended testing only when there are features present in the history or examination that suggest bleeding disorders (grade C recommendation). In contrast, the American College of Obstetricians and Gynecologists guidelines of 2001)[24] recommend screening for von Willebrand's disease in all adolescents with menorrhagia, as well as all adults with no pelvic pathology and in all women prior to hysterectomy.

Taking a good history of bleeding is important in identifying women who are more likely to have von Willebrand's disease. In history taking, the duration of menorrhagia and any history of post-partum haemorrhage, postoperative haemorrhage and bleeding after dental extraction should be checked. We found in our population that menorrhagia since menarche was present in 65% of women who were subsequently diagnosed to have von Willebrand's disease compared to 9% in the rest.[19] The prevalence of post-partum haemorrhage, postoperative bleeding and bleeding after dental extraction were significantly higher in women who were diagnosed to have von Willebrand's disease.[19] Therefore, there should be a high index of suspicion of a bleeding disorder in women with long-standing menorrhagia and history of bleeding after haemostatic challenge. However, over 50% of women diagnosed to have bleeding disorders by Dilley et al.[20] suffered no other bleeding symptoms. Thus, the clinical severity of von Willebrand's disease varies considerably, and menorrhagia may be the only clinical manifestation. Hence, the argument for testing all patients with menorrhagia.

In addition to von Willebrand's disease, other bleeding disorders can be the underlying cause for menorrhagia. FXI deficiency was found in our centre in 4% (6/150) of patients with menorrhagia.[19] Interestingly, only 2 of the 6 women were of Jewish origin. von Willebrand's Factor was significantly lower in these women compared to those without bleeding disorders and two of the women had combined von Willebrand's disease/FXI deficiency. The prevalence of platelet defects as well as fibrinolytic disorders in women with menorrhagia is presently unknown. Recently Philipp et al.[25] found abnormal platelet aggregation and decreased platelet ATP release in 47% and 56% of 70 women with menorrhagia, respectively. Prolonged closure time was also reported in 29% of cases using Platelet Function Analyser (PFA–100). Therefore, testing for these disorders is worth considering in unexplained menorrhagia with normal von Willebrand's Factor levels, especially in patients with other bleeding symptoms.

Undiagnosed thrombocytopenia has not been shown to be an underlying cause for menorrhagia in adults. In contrast, it seems to be a common cause of adolescent menorrhagia.[17,26] Thrombocytopenia (platelet count $< 150,000/\mu l$) has been reported in 13% of 71 girls aged 10–19 years with menorrhagia,[26] including three newly diagnosed ITP. In the same study, 14 of the 71 girls underwent a more detailed haemostatic evaluation and platelet function defects were diagnosed in 6 and type 1 von Willebrand's disease in 2 of the girls. Platelet disorders cause other bleeding symptoms, in particular bruising and petechiae and epistaxis, thus earlier presentation and diagnosis. In addition, acute thrombocytopenia is more common in this age group.

Diagnosis of inherited bleeding disorders in women with menorrhagia has several medical implications. First, it enhances rapid and effective treatment of menorrhagia. Second, if any surgical intervention becomes necessary, the risk of bleeding complications can be minimized by appropriate pre-operative assessment and prophylactic treatment when indicated. Lastly, it has genetic ramifications and important implications for the management of any future pregnancies.

DIAGNOSIS OF MENORRHAGIA AND VON WILLEBRAND'S DISEASE

There are some debatable issues in the diagnosis of menorrhagia and inherited bleeding disorders, in particular von Willebrand's disease, worth considering further.

von Willebrand's disease

Diagnosis of von Willebrand's disease is difficult and there is a debate as to which test should be used for screening of patients with menorrhagia. In the absence of genetic analysis, the diagnosis of von Willebrand's disease is made on a clinical basis and on laboratory results of coagulation screen and clotting factor (von Willebrand's Factor:Ag [vWF:Ag], von Willebrand's Factor:Ac [vWF:Ac], Factor VIII activity [FVIII:C]) assays. However, the clinical expression of the disease is variable and the laboratory data may overlap with the normal range and fluctuate with time in a given individual making the diagnosis, especially of mild forms, difficult and complex. Bleeding time and APTT are usually prolonged in patients with von Willebrand's disease. However, these tests may be normal in most of the patients with mild disease and may, therefore, not be sensitive enough to be used for screening and diagnosis of this disorder. The APTT reflects deficiencies of Factors VIII, IX, XI and XII; but, when the concentration of these factors are over 30% of normal, the APTT will not be prolonged. In patients with mild von Willebrand's disease, FVIII:C, vWF:Ag, vWF:Ac levels are variable and may be normal, but on repeated testing at least one abnormal value is usually observed. The vWF:Ac assay is the single most sensitive assay for screening for most forms of von Willebrand's disease. Because of the variability of laboratory findings in von Willebrand's disease, repeated testing to establish the diagnosis of mild von Willebrand's disease is recommended especially with borderline levels.

There is a large intra-individual variation in von Willebrand's Factor and Factor VIII levels, especially in women as these factors fluctuate during the menstrual cycle.[27] The restriction of sampling to the early follicular phase of the cycle, when the levels are at their baseline, has been suggested to minimise this variation. However, from personal experience, the best time to do the first test is at presentation as some women may not return for the test, and the last menstrual period should be noted. However, subsequent tests because of borderline values should be done between days 1–7 of the cycle.

There is also concern about concurrent use of combined oral contraceptives when testing for von Willebrand's disease. Oestradiol has been shown to increase levels of von Willebrand's Factor and there have been some reports where diagnosis of von Willebrand's disease was obscured in women on the pill. However, the current combined oral contraceptives have low oestradiol levels (30 µg oestradiol) and Factor VIII, vWF:Ag and vWF:Ac were reported not to be statistically different in women taking these compared to non-pill users.[27]

Factor VIII and von Willebrand's Factor have been shown to be significantly lower in individuals with type O blood group compared to non-O. Therefore, adjustment for ABO blood type has been suggested. However, Nitu-Whalley *et al.*[28] reviewed 246 patients with type 1 von Willebrand's disease and showed that 70% of the patients were blood group O. The bleeding symptoms were similar in O and non-O individuals with von Willebrand's disease Factor levels of 35–50 IU/dl. Therefore, we conclude that von Willebrand's disease is common in individuals with blood group O and the clinical picture is the same regardless of the blood group. Factor VIII and von Willebrand's Factor are also significantly higher in Afro-Caribbeans compared to those of other ethnic origins.[27] Recently, Miller *et al.*[29] showed that using different ranges for Afro-Caribbean could improve the detection rate of von Willebrand's disease.

Menorrhagia

The diagnosis of menorrhagia is also difficult and usually subjectively based on a patient's description of menstrual loss. Although the patient's impression is an important issue when managing menorrhagia, it is unfortunately an inaccurate assessment and there is lack of correlation with actual menstrual blood loss. Haemoglobin determination of menstrual blood, using the alkaline haematin method as described by Hallberg and Nilsson,[30] is currently the most reliable technique and has been widely used in many studies. However, the method is expensive, time-consuming and inconvenient to the patients, and, as such, is not practical for everyday use in clinical practice.

The pictorial blood assessment chart (PBAC) has been introduced as a simple, non-laboratory method for semi-quantitative measure of menstrual blood loss. Using a score of > 100 as equivalent to a menstrual loss of > 80 ml, the PBAC was shown to have a reasonable accuracy with a sensitivity of 86% and a specificity of 89% compared with the alkaline haematin method.[4] Janssen *et al.*[5] re-validated the chart but suggested a score of 185 as a cut-off point to maximise its predictive values. However, a score of 185 has a much lower sensitivity and negative predictive value compared to a score of 100. The PBAC is a screening tool to help the diagnosis of menorrhagia and guide patient response to treatment. Therefore, a cut-off point with a higher sensitivity is much more appropriate than one with high specificity and positive predictive value with which diagnosis of some borderline cases can be overlooked. On the other hand, Reid *et al.*[31] cast doubt on the validity of the chart and found poor correlation between the PBAC score and menstrual blood loss.

MANAGEMENT OF MENORRHAGIA

Menorrhagia in women with inherited bleeding disorders is likely to be due to the clotting factor deficiency, but not exclusively. Therefore, each individual should be appropriately assessed and local causes excluded especially the possibility of malignancy in older women. Close collaboration with haematologists is important and ideally these patients should be managed in a joint haematology and gynaecology clinic.

MEDICAL TREATMENT

The treatment of menorrhagia is usually medical and the most commonly used, first-line options are tranexamic acid, combined oral contraceptive compounds, or more recently intra-nasal DDAVP spray. The choice is dependent on the patient's age, reproductive state and preference and availability of the medications, as well as the clinician's experience and preference.

Tranexamic acid

Antifibrinolytic agents have a beneficial role in the management of menorrhagia as fibrinolytic activity increases during menstruation. Tranexamic acid significantly reduces endometrial tissue plasminogen activator activity and antigen and reduces menstrual blood loss in patients with menorrhagia in general, as well as in patients with inherited bleeding disorders. Bonnar and Sheppard[32] randomised 76 women to one of three treatments: (i) ethamsylate (a general haemostatic agent); (ii) mefenamic acid (a prostaglandin synthetase inhibitor); and (iii) the fibrinolytic agent, tranexamic acid at a dose of 1 g 6 hourly. Menstrual loss measured by the spectrophotometric method in three control menstrual periods and three menstrual periods during treatment showed that there was no reduction in menstrual blood loss with ethamsylate, a 20% reduction with mefenamic acid, and a 54% reduction with tranexamic acid. The side-effects of tranexamic acid included nausea, headache and dizziness, but 77% of the women were happy to continue the treatment. There has been some concern about its thrombotic complications, although a recent study showed no increased risk of thrombosis in women.[33] Tranexamic acid is effective, safe and far less expensive than other treatment modalities and should be considered as a first-line therapy. The bioavailability of tranexamic acid is only about 35%, which requires administration of at least 1 g 4–6 hourly necessary which may reduce patient compliance. There is a recent report of the successful use of single high-dose antifibrinolytic therapy (tranexamic acid at a dose of 4 g orally) in three type 2A and 2B von Willebrand's disease.[34] However, in our experience, this dosage is associated with severe nausea and vomiting.

Combined oral contraceptives

Combined oral contraceptives (OCPs) control menstrual cycle and inhibit endometrial growth as well as increasing FVIII:C and vWF:Ac levels. Therefore, it is commonly used for patients with inherited bleeding disorders and menorrhagia. However, there was no demonstrable increase in Factor VIII and von Willebrand's Factor with the use of low dose (30 µg oestradiol) pills.[2] In addition, their efficacy in reducing the menstrual loss in women with von Willebrand's disease or other bleeding disorders is unknown. In a survey of type 2 and 3 von Willebrand's disease patients by Foster et al.,[12] 88% of women treated with OCPs stated they were effective. In another study in type 1 von Willebrand's disease patients, a standard dose of OCPs was effective 24% of the time and high-dose oral contraceptive therapy was effective only 37% of the time.[6] OCPs have added benefit of regular menstrual cycles and reliable contraception. On the other hand, OCPs are associated with risk of thrombosis, but women with bleeding disorders have a low inherited thrombotic risk.

DDAVP (desmopressin) nasal spray

DDAVP (1-deamino-8-D-arginine vasopressin), a vasopressin analogue, has an established role in the management of patients with type 1 von Willebrand's disease and mild-to-moderate haemophilia A due to its ability to cause an increase in plasma concentrations of Factor VIII and von Willebrand's Factor. Patients with type 2A von Willebrand's disease may also respond to DDAVP. In type 2B von Willebrand's disease, a rare subtype, DDAVP may induce thrombocytopenia and may, therefore, be contra-indicated for the management of these patients. Effective and safe use has been shown in selected clinical situations in these patients, but most clinicians are reluctant to use it. Patients with type 3 von Willebrand's disease do not respond to DDAVP. DDAVP is currently regarded as an important therapeutic alternative to plasma-derived coagulation products in selected cases because of efficacy and no risk of infection with blood-borne viruses. A test dose is usually performed prior to treatment to differentiate responders from non-responders.

Several formulations of DDAVP are available, including intravenous infusion, subcutaneous injection and a highly concentrated intranasal spray, which is ideal for home use. Clinical effectiveness of the spray has also been demonstrated in reducing bleeding symptoms when used at home. The use of plasma products is reduced, as well as the number of visits to out-patient clinics and absence from school or work with this home treatment. Side effects of DDAVP are very few, usually mild tachycardia, headache and flushing due to the vasomotor effects. There is also a slight risk of hyponatraemia and, potentially, water intoxication as DDAVP has an antidiuretic effect. This complication can be greatly reduced by strict fluid restriction and electrolyte monitoring, especially in those receiving several doses of DDAVP.

Kobrinsky and Goldsmith[35] conducted a multicentre prospective trial using DDAVP nasal spray for treatment of menorrhagia in 68 patients with type 1 von Willebrand's disease and 15 carriers of haemophilia A. An interactive, voice-response technology system was used to register whether the treatment was effective (excellent or good response) or had minimal or no response. The efficacy was assessed daily and among 552 and 151 daily ratings, response was considered effective in 92% and 95% of the time in von Willebrand's disease patients and carriers of haemophilia, respectively.

Despite the apparent efficacy for home use of DDAVP nasal spray, objective data on menstrual loss were not examined. We have recently performed a randomised, placebo-controlled, cross-over study using PBAC for assessment of menstrual blood loss. There was significant decrease in PBAC scores with DDAVP and with placebo compared to pre-treatment. The menstrual blood loss was also reduced with DDAVP compared to placebo, but the difference was not statistically significant. We also found a significant decrease in menstrual blood loss throughout the trial and the scores were significantly lower during the second treatment period, which also indicates the placebo effect.[36]

At present, there is no consensus regarding the dose and duration of DDAVP spray for treatment of menorrhagia. It is usually given in the first 2–3 days of the period based on the findings that 90% of all menstrual flow is in the first 3 days.[5] However, in women with bleeding disorders, we have shown that these women bleed heavily throughout their menstruation.[2] Therefore, dose and duration should be tailored according to the PBAC assessment. Considering the efficacy of combined therapy in the management of mucosal bleeding in patients with inherited bleeding disorders, using a combination treatment of DDAVP spray and antifibrinolytics needs to be explored for the management of menorrhagia.

Other medical treatments
Progestogens are widely used in the treatment of dysfunctional uterine bleeding despite the limited evidence to support their ability to decrease menstrual blood loss. In high doses, oral progestogens or in the form of Depot Provera, alone or in combination with DDAVP or factor concentrate may be useful to arrest acute haemorrhage. Cyclical progestogens are only effective if used from Day 5 to Day 26 of the cycle. This can be considered as a second line treatment for women with bleeding disorders and menorrhagia who do not respond to the first line treatment or when it is contraindicate. Luteal phase treatment with progestogen is ineffective in the treatment of menorrhagia.

Other medical treatments including danazol and gonadotropin releasing hormone agonists are effective in the treatment of menorrhagia. However, they have a high incidence of side effects, are expensive and cannot be used for long-term treatment.

LEVONORGESTREL INTRA-UTERINE SYSTEM, MIRENA (LNG IUS)

Levonorgestrel intra-uterine system, Mirena (LNG IUS) has been shown to be highly effective in reducing menstrual loss in premenopausal women. In a recent systematic review of five randomised controlled trials and five case series, menstrual blood loss was reduced by 74–97% at 3 and 12 months, and 65–80% of patients on the waiting list for hysterectomy were taken off after using the Levonorgestrel intra-uterine system.[37] After a year of follow-up, quality-of-life and psychological well-being have been reported to be equal to hysterectomy in a randomised trial by Hurskainen et al.[38] The main problem with Mirena is a high discontinuation rate at 20% in randomised controlled trials, and 17% in case series reviewed by Stewart et al.[37] because of irregular bleeding during the first 3–6 months and progestogenic side effects. Proper counselling and patient education may increase tolerance. This method is widely used especially prior to a decision on surgical management. The Levonorgestrel intra-uterine system is an effective and reversible method of contraception, which is an added advantage in women who wish to preserve their fertility.

Due to the high local level of progestogen, the use of the hormone-releasing system results in endometrial suppression. In addition this intra-uterine system has no effect on endometrial Factor VIII activity, which is reduced by intra-uterine contraceptive devices.[39] We are currently evaluating the Levonorgestrel intra-uterine system for management of menorrhagia in bleeding disorders.

SURGICAL MANAGEMENT

Surgical intervention may be required in patients unresponsive to medical treatment. Even relatively minor operations, such as hysteroscopy and/or diagnostic curettage, can be complicated by haemorrhage in patients with inherited bleeding disorders. Good liaison between the local haemophilia centre and the surgical/anaesthetic team is essential. Clotting factor levels should be checked pre-operatively and adequate haemostatic cover provided to maintain the levels at > 50 IU/dl and > 30 IU/dl for major and minor surgery, respectively, until healing is complete. Therefore, the treatment may need to be continued postoperatively, possibly up to 10 days, to prevent secondary bleeding and haematomas. Surgical interventions should be carried out by an experienced gynaecologist using a technique with least risk of bleeding. Bleeding vessels should be ligated and not cauterised as oozing can occur after surgery. Surgical drains should be onsidered. It is also important to remember that excessive bleeding may be surgical and not due to failure of adequate replacement therapy. Depending on the nature of the operation and the clotting factor levels, monitoring postoperatively is continued. Secondary haemorrhage at 7–10 days is not uncommon and, following major surgery, in-patient observation may be necessary for this length of time. Likewise, any unexplained operative and postoperative bleeding that does not respond to general measures should alert the gynaecologist to the possibility of a bleeding disorders.

Hysterectomy is the definitive treatment with the highest patient satisfaction, but is a major operation associated with a mortality of 3/10,000 and 3% serious morbidity.[40] Endometrial ablative techniques are increasingly used for management of menorrhagia not responding to medical treatment. Endometrial ablation is associated with shorter operative time, fewer complications and faster return to normal activity and work. Endometrial resection carries a risk of bleeding complications and thermal or laser ablation are advised in patients with bleeding disorders. More recently, several non-hysteroscopic techniques (microwave endometrial ablation, thermal balloon ablation, hydrothermal ablation, cryo-ablation and others) have been introduced in an attempt to find simple, quicker and safer procedures that can be used in the out-patient setting. Data regarding the performance of these procedures are still lacking. Hopefully this evidence will soon be available from randomised trials which are currently in progress.

Key points for clinical practice

- Menorrhagia in a significant proportion of women diagnosed as dysfunctional uterine bleeding is due to undiagnosed bleeding disorders, especially von Willebrand's disease.

- Testing for von Willebrand's disease should be part of the investigation for women with menorrhagia before embarking on any surgical intervention for diagnosis or treatment.

- Detailed bleeding history is crucial to identify women requiring investigation for bleeding disorders.

Key points for clinical practice (continued)

- Close collaboration with haematologists is required in the management of women with menorrhagia, when a bleeding disorder is suspected or diagnosed.

- Women with bleeding disorders suffer significant gynaecological morbidity, including menorrhagia, dysmenorrhea and mid-cycle pain that can affect their health and quality-of-life.

- Increased awareness among clinicians of these problems and treatment options available is essential to improve quality of life. Tranexamic acid is a safe, effective and inexpensive treatment for menorrhagia in these women and should be used as first-line management.

- DDAVP nasal spray increases von Willebrand's Factor and Factor VIII levels and can be used as a home treatment for some women with bleeding disorders. A test dose is required to assess response.

- The Levonorgestrel intra-uterine system should be considered prior to surgery.

- A multidisciplinary team approach is required when contemplating gynaecological surgery in these women to minimise bleeding complications.

References

1. Christiaens GC, Sixma JJ, Haspels AA. Morphology of haemostasis in menstrual endometrium. *Br J Obstet Gynaecol* 1980; **87**: 425–439.
2. Kadir RA, Economides DL, Sabin CA, Pollard D, Lee CA. Assessment of menstrual blood loss and gynaecological problems in patients with inherited bleeding disorders. *Haemophilia* 1999; **5**: 40–48.
3. von Willebrand EA. Hereditary pseudohamofili. *Finnska Iaekaellsk handl* 1926; **68**: 87–112.
4. Higham JM, O'Brien PM, Shaw RW. Assessment of menstrual blood loss using a pictorial chart. *Br J Obstet Gynaecol* 1990; **97**: 734–739.
5. Janssen CA, Scholten PC, Heintz AP. A simple visual assessment technique to discriminate between menorrhagia and normal menstrual blood loss. *Obstet Gynecol* 1995; **85**: 977–982.
6. Kouides P, Phatak P, Burkhart P *et al*. Gynaecological and obstetrical morbidity in women with type 1 von Willebrand disease: results of a patient survey. *Haemophilia* 2000; **6**: 643–648.
7. Ragni M, Bontempo F, Cortese Hassett A. von Willebrand disease and bleeding in women. *Haemophilia* 1999; **5**: 313–317.
8. Lusher JM, McMillan CW. Severe factor VIII and factor IX deficiency in females. *Am J Med* 1978; **65**: 637–648.
9. Mauser Bunschoten EP, van Houwelingen JC, van Sjamsoedin Visser EJ *et al*. Bleeding symptoms in carriers of hemophilia A and B. *Thromb Haemost* 1988; **59**: 349–352.
10. Bolton-Maggs PH, Patterson DA, Wensley RT, Tuddenham EG. Definition of the bleeding tendency in factor XI-deficient kindreds – a clinical and laboratory study. *Thromb Haemost* 1995; **73**: 194–202.
11. Rozeik Ch, Scharrer I. Gynecological disorders and psychological problems in 184 women with von Willebrand disease. *Haemophilia* 1998; **4**: 293.

12. Foster PA. The reproductive health of women with von Willebrand disease unresponsive to DDAVP: results of an international survey. On behalf of the Subcommittee on von Willebrand Factor of the Scientific and Standardization Committee of the ISTH. *Thromb Haemost* 1995; **74**: 784–790.

13. Kadir RA, Sabin CA, Pollard D, Lee CA, Economides DL. Quality of life during menstruation in patients with inherited bleeding disorders. *Haemophilia* 1998; **4**: 836–841.

14. Gomez A, Lucia JF, Perella M, Aguilar C. Haemoperitoneum caused by haemorrhagic corpus luteum in a patient with type 3 von Willebrand's disease. *Haemophilia* 1998; **4**: 60–62.

15. Greer IA, Lowe GD, Walker JJ, Forbes CD. Haemorrhagic problems in obstetrics and gynaecology in patients with congenital coagulopathies. *Br J Obstet Gynaecol* 1991; **98**: 909–918.

16. Edlund M, Magnusson C, Von Schoultz B. Quality of life – a Swedish survey of 2200 women. In: Smith SK. (ed) *Dysfunctional Uterine Bleeding*. London: The Royal Society of Medicine Press, 1994; XX–XX.

17. Claessens EA, Cowell CA. Acute adolescent menorrhagia. *Am J Obstet Gynecol* 1981; **139**: 277–280.

18. Edlund M, Blomback M, von Schoultz B, Andersson O. On the value of menorrhagia as a predictor for coagulation disorders. *Am J Hematol* 1996; **53**: 234–238.

19. Kadir RA, Economides DL, Sabin CA, Owens D, Lee CA. Frequency of inherited bleeding disorders in women with menorrhagia. *Lancet* 1998; **351**: 485–489.

20. Dilley A, Drews C, Miller C *et al.* von Willebrand disease and other inherited bleeding disorders in women with diagnosed menorrhagia. *Obstet Gynecol* 2001; **97**: 630–636.

21. Woo Y, White B, Corbally R *et al.* von Willebrand disease: an important cause of dysfunctional uterine bleeding. *Blood Coagul Fibrinolysis* 2002; **13**: 89–93.

22. Werner EJ, Broxson EH, Tucker EL, Giroux DS, Shults J, Abshire TC. Prevalence of von Willebrand disease in children: a multiethnic study. *J Pediatr* 1993; **123**: 893–898.

23. Anon. *The Initial Management of Menorrhagia. Evidence-based Clinical Guidelines No. 1.* London: The Royal College of Obstetricians and Gynaecologists, 1998.

24. Anon. *von Willebrand's Disease in Gynecologic Practice.* Committee opinion No 263. *American College of Obstetricians and Gynecologists* 2001; **98**: 1185–1186.

25. Philipp CS, Dilley A, Miller CH, Evatt B, Saidi P. Platelet defects in women with unexplained menorrhagia [Abstract]. *Haemophilia* 2002; **8**: 512.

26. Bevan JA, Maloney KW, Gill JC, Montgomery RR, Scott JP. Bleeding cause of menorrhagia in adolescents. *J Pediatr* 2001; **138**: 856–861.

27. Kadir RA, Economides DL, Sabin CA, Owens D, Lee CA. Variations in coagulation factors in women: effect of age, ethnicity, menstrual cycle and combined oral contraceptive. *Thromb Haemost* 1999; **82**: 1456–1461.

28. Nitu-Whalley J, Lee CA, Griffioen A, Jenkins PV, Pasi KJ. Type 1 von Willebrand disease – a clinical retrospective study of diagnosis, the influence of ABO blood group and the role of bleeding history. *Br J Haematol* 2000; **108**: 259–264.

29. Miller Ch, Dilley A, Richardson L, Hooper WC, Evatt BL. Population differences in von Willebrand factor levels affects diagnosis of von Willebrand disease in African American women. *Am J Hematol* 2001; **67**: 125–129.

30. Hallberg L, Nilsson L. Determination of menstrual blood loss. *Scand J Clin Lab Invest* 1964; **16**: 244–248.

31. Reid P, Coker A, Ciltart R. Assessment of menstrual loss using a pictorial blood chart: a validation study. *Br J Obstet Gynaecol* 2000; **107**: 320–322.

32. Bonnar J, Sheppard BL. Treatment of menorrhagia during menstruation: randomised controlled trial of ethamsylate, mefenamic acid, and tranexamic acid. *BMJ* 1996; **313**: 579–582.

33. Berntorp E, Follrud C, Lethagen S. No increased risk of venous thrombosis in women taking tranexamic acid. *Thromb Haemost* 2001; **86**: 714–715.

34. Ong YL, Hull DR, Mayne EE. Menorrhagia in von Willebrand disease successfully treated with single daily dose tranexamic acid. *Haemophilia* 1998; **4**: 63–65.

35. Kobrinsky N, Goldsmith J. Efficacy of Stimate (desmopressin acetate) nasal spray, 1.5 mg/ml, for the treatment of menorrhagia in women with inherited bleeding disorders [Abstract]. *Blood* 1997; **90 (Suppl 1)**: 106.

36. Kadir RA, Lee CA, Pollard D, Economides DL. DDAVP nasal spray for treatment of menorrhagia in women with inherited bleeding disorders: a randomised placebo controlled cross-over study. *Haemophilia* 2002; In press.
37. Stewart A, Cummins, Gold L, Jordan R, Phillips W. The effectiveness of the levonorgestrel-releasing intra-uterine system in menorrhagia: a systematic review. *Br J Obstet Gynaecol* 2001; **108**: 74–86.
38. Hurskainen R, Teperi J, Aalto S *et al*. Quality of life and cost-effectiveness of the levonorgestrel-releasing intra-uterine system versus hysterectomy for treatment of menorrhagia: a randomised trial. *Lancet* 2001: **357**: 273–277.
39. Zhu P, Hongzhi L, Wenliang S. Observation of the activity of factor VIII in the endometrium of women pre- and post-insertion of three types of IUDs. *Contraception* 1991; **44**: 367–387.
40. Maresh M, Metcalfe M, McPherson K. The VALUE national hysterectomy study: description of patients and their surgery. *Br J Obstet Gynaecol* 2002; **109**: 302–312.

David E. Parkin Stuart Jack

10

Evidence-based surgical treatment for dysfunctional uterine bleeding

Until the introduction of the first generation, hysteroscopic methods of endometrial laser ablation (ELA) and transcervical resection of the endometrium (TCRE) in the late 1980s, a hysterectomy was the only definitive surgical treatment for dysfunctional uterine bleeding (DUB). Despite hysterectomy being very common, there was little hard evidence regarding its role. The new endometrial ablative methods (including resection) gave the promise of replacing hysterectomy with a minor, quick, and safe technique.

The early 1990s was a time when the concept of evidence-based medicine was becoming established. This meant that the newly introduced endometrial ablative methods were rigorously assessed with randomised controlled trials comparing them to hysterectomy, medical treatment and the differing methods of ablation. As a result, evidence regarding all the surgical methods including hysterectomy began to accrue. At the same time, national audits of endometrial ablation, and recently hysterectomy gave robust data regarding safety.

Despite the increasing acceptance of the role of randomised trials, it is unfortunate that the majority of publications in this area are uncontrolled observational studies. Furthermore, only the minority of studies have used power calculations to determine the size of the population studied.

Outcome measures are a problem with studies on surgery for DUB. Patient satisfaction is the most useful and important measure, followed by hysterectomy rates following ablative surgery. Amenorrhoea rates are useful when comparing one ablative method with another, but less so when comparing ablation to hysterectomy. Surrogate measures of menstrual loss are even less useful as even the PBLAC score has been shown to be unreliable in women with DUB.[1]

David E. Parkin MD FRCOG, Consultant Gynaecologist, Department of Gynaecology, Aberdeen Royal Infirmary, Forresterhill, Aberdeen AB25 2ZN, UK (for correspondence)

Stuart Jack MRCOG, Specialist Registrar, Department of Gynaecology, Aberdeen Royal Infirmary, Forresterhill, Aberdeen AB25 2ZN, UK

Patient selection for trials and studies is another area where bias is possible. A number of prognostic factors for the success or failure of endometrial ablation have been recognised. Success is more likely in women who are older, have genuinely heavy periods and who have less dysmenorrhoea.[2] Studies can, therefore, be biased if the population is not representative. Care must be taken when interpreting results of studies, especially those that are not randomised or have inclusion and exclusion criteria based on PBLAC scores.

The main areas for discussion are: (i) when to offer surgical treatment for DUB; (ii) hysterectomy or endometrial ablation – results and safety; (iii) patient selection for endometrial ablation; and (iv) which method of endometrial ablation.

WHEN TO OFFER SURGICAL TREATMENT FOR DUB

When hysterectomy was the only surgical method for the treatment of DUB, it was seldom employed as a first line treatment before trying multiple medical treatments and repeated uterine curettage. Only when these failed was a hysterectomy considered. This was sensible as hysterectomy is a major procedure not without risks. As the endometrial ablative methods were thought of as an alternative to hysterectomy, the same view was held.

All the surgical methods, hysterectomy and ablation should only be offered to women who have completed their family. The only data regarding the place of medical *versus* primary surgical treatment for DUB come from a randomised trial comparing oral medical treatment with TCRE and from some trials of the Levonorgestrel IUS (Mirena).

Cooper *et al.* randomised patients referred for the first time to a gynaecological clinic to either medical (oral) treatment or TCRE.[3,4] The study was pragmatic in design and adequately powered. At 5 years, women allocated to medical treatment were significantly less likely to be totally satisfied or to recommend their treatment to a friend despite the majority ultimately receiving either a TCRE or hysterectomy. Bleeding and pain scores were similar in both groups and significantly reduced in both compared to the pre-treatment levels. In the TCRE arm, significantly more women had no or very light bleeding and significantly fewer days of heavy bleeding. The hysterectomy rates at 5 years for the two arms were very similar (18% in the medical arm and 20% in the TCRE arm).

TCRE improved quality-of-life as measured by all 8 health scales of the Short Form 36 compared to only 4 after medical treatment, and restored them to normative levels. TCRE achieved higher levels of satisfaction, better menstrual status, and a greater improvement in health-related quality-of-life without an increase in the hysterectomy rate. The study predated the licensed use of the Mirena (Levonorgestrel IUS) in DUB.

A number of RCTs exist comparing Mirena to surgical management. An Italian study randomised 70 women referred for hysterectomy in a 1:1 ratio to either insertion of a Mirena or TCRE.[5] Follow-up was up to 1 year with the main outcome measures being menstrual bleeding, patient satisfaction and quality-of-life. Amenorrhoea or hypomenorrhoea was significantly higher after TCRE (71%) than after Mirena (65%). There was no statistically significant difference in the satisfaction rate, 94% with TCRE and 85% with Mirena, or quality-of-life. The small numbers and the invalidation of the power study are concerns with this report.

Mirena has been compared to hysterectomy in two Finnish randomised controlled trials (RCTs). The first trial randomised 56 women on a waiting list for hysterectomy to either continuing their current medical treatment or to Mirena.[6] By 6 months, 64.3% in the Mirena Group had cancelled their hysterectomy compared to 14.3% in the control arm. By 12 months, half of the women in the Mirena arm had a hysterectomy. Just under half (48%) were still using their Mirena at 3 years. Though these results are encouraging, certain problems in interpretation of the study results exist. The study did not recruit enough patients to reach statistical power as the ethical committee halted the study when the waiting time for hysterectomy fell. Secondly, as these women were on a long waiting list for hysterectomy, their involvement in the study may have been biased by a 'nothing-to-lose' factor.

In the second Finnish multicentre study, 236 women were randomised to Mirena or hysterectomy.[7] In the Mirena arm, one-third of the patients had their devices removed mainly for inter-menstrual bleeding, and 20% underwent hysterectomy in the first year. The authors concluded that health-related quality-of-life (and other indices of psychological health) improved significantly in both groups, that patients in the hysterectomy group suffered significantly less pain, and that overall costs at 1 year were 3 times higher for hysterectomy than Mirena.

Mirena does have a place and may replace either endometrial ablation or hysterectomy in a number of cases. It is especially useful when there is uncertainty over future fertility wishes. When comparing TCRE to Mirena, no study has been of sufficient size for adequate assessment. TCRE offers a significantly greater reduction in menstrual loss and a higher amenorrhoea rate than Mirena.

HYSTERECTOMY OR ENDOMETRIAL ABLATION – RESULTS AND SAFETY

RESULTS

When TCRE and ELA were introduced into the UK, a number of randomised trials were carried out comparing these new techniques to hysterectomy. As the complaint of DUB is subjective and selection criteria for surgery vary, it was essential to perform RCTs to compare endometrial ablation to hysterectomy.

Four RCTs have been published which differ in their methodological soundness and also the length of follow-up. Gannon et al. published the first study;[8] 51 women who were already on the waiting list for hysterectomy were randomised in a 1:1 ratio between hysterectomy or TCRE and were followed for 9 months postoperatively. Dwyer et al. randomised 200 women to either hysterectomy or TCRE (ratio 1:1) at the time of the decision to offer surgical treatment for their heavy periods and follow-up was for 2 years.[9] Pinion et al. randomised 204 women to either hysterectomy or hysteroscopic surgery (1:1 ratio).[10] Follow-up has now been published at 4–6 years postoperatively.[11] O'Connor published an MRC funded multicentre study.[12] Unfortunately, this study used a 3:1 randomisation between TCRE and hysterectomy, had a prolonged period of recruitment, and 75% of eligible women declined to enter the study. It was a multicentre study and the results were perhaps more generally applicable than the single centre studies above. Despite the methodological differences between these studies, the results are remarkably consistent.

In the Dwyer study, satisfaction after TCRE was 84% compared to 93% with hysterectomy.[9] After 12 months' follow up, Pinion found 78% of women were satisfied with the result of TCRE/ELA and 89% satisfied after hysterectomy.[10] O'Connor found 85% satisfaction after TCRE compared to 96% after hysterectomy at a median follow-up of 2 years though the validity of the hysterectomy results are reduced by the fact that there were only 28 women in the hysterectomy group.[12] All three studies showed significantly shorter recovery time, shorter hospital stay, and significantly fewer complications after endometrial ablation compared to hysterectomy.

These studies confirmed the previous observational findings that hysterectomy does not lead to 100% patient satisfaction when carried out for excessive menstrual loss despite giving complete amenorrhoea.

These studies were pragmatic and included women with uterine enlargement up to the size of a 10-week pregnancy and 20% had fibroids identifiable at hysteroscopy. In the hysterectomy group, endometriosis was found in 8% and adenomyosis in 17% of the women so it can be assumed that the women in the TCRE group had similar pathology.[10] This meant that the women in these studies had not been carefully selected to include only women with no pathology and regular uterine cavities.

Long-term follow-up of the Pinion study from Aberdeen has been published.[11] The follow-up period was 4–6 years with a median of 5.1 years. Hysterectomy was avoided in 76% of the hysteroscopic surgery group. There was no significant difference in satisfaction between the two groups. Life table analysis showed that hysterectomy was only seldom needed once women were beyond 36 months after their hysteroscopic surgery. This result is re-assuring and shows that hysterectomy was avoided in three-quarters of this group of women. This was despite the fact that these women were expecting a hysterectomy and associated amenorrhoea.

Persistence of pelvic pain following endometrial ablation is a common reason for apparent failure of the technique and the cause of subsequent hysterectomy. In the Aberdeen study, 15% of women continued to suffer from pelvic pain 4–6 years after hysterectomy compared to 18% after hysteroscopic surgery. If abdominal or pelvic pain continues following endometrial ablation pain, it is often managed by hysterectomy.

The relative symptomatic results of the two treatment approaches are best assessed by the use of RCTs as shown above. These are large enough to give an indication of the relative frequency of common complications, but for the study of uncommon complications large prospective series are needed. Fortunately two such audits of the hysteroscopic methods have been carried out in the UK and recently one on the complications of hysterectomy.

SAFETY

Complications of endometrial resection and ablation

The incidence of complications following the hysteroscopic methods of TCRE and ELA were first investigated by the Scottish Audit of Hysteroscopic

Surgery[13] and then by the MISTLETOE study in England and Wales.[14] These studies between them give the results in over 11,000 patients. Both audits estimated that over 90% of procedures were reported and that there was no difference in the complication rate in the unreported group. In the MISTLETOE study of over 10,000 cases, the rate of bowel damage due to TCRE was 7/10,000.[14] The Scottish Audit of Hysteroscopy Surgery study of just under 1000 patients reported no cases of bowel damage. However, one case, which was reported to the audit as a uterine perforation and laparoscopy following TCRE, was actually a case of small bowel damage. The patient subsequently required a laparotomy after the registration form was returned.[13] This gives a rate of 1/1000 for bowel damage due to TCRE. Endometrial laser ablation (ELA) may be safer than TCRE with no case of bowel damage in 1764 cases in MISTLETOE and 314 in the Scottish audit, but there was a case of small bowel damage in the Aberdeen randomised study.[10]

Rollerball endometrial ablation (REA) is a first-generation method derived from TCRE and felt to be a safer method as the surface of the uterine cavity is coagulated rather than resected. No visceral damage was reported with this method in MISTLETOE, but there were only 650 cases.[14] There have been a number of case reports of large and small bowel damage after REA. In the MISTLETOE study, the rate of emergency hysterectomy was 6/1000 overall, but 11/1000 when TCRE was performed using a loop for the whole procedure. In the Scottish audit, the emergency hysterectomy rate was 2/1000, considerably lower than the English audit. Uterine perforation was reported in 15/1000 cases in the MISTLETOE and 10/1000 in the Scottish audit.[13,14] This is of little consequence provided the perforation is recognised and does not involve the use of electrodiathermy or laser energy.

As all the hysteroscopic methods use fluid to distend and irrigate the uterine cavity, excessive absorption of irrigation fluid is a potential risk. During TCRE using glycine, changes in electrolytes especially serum sodium can be avoided if the procedure is abandoned when absorption is noted to be reaching 1500 ml. In MISTLETOE, there was a 1% rate of fluid absorption of greater than 2000 ml and 1% in the Scottish audit. Both audits and a RCT comparing TCRE to ELA have shown a greater rate of fluid absorption following ELA as compared to TCRE.[13–15] Combining the two audit studies, the mortality from the hysteroscopic methods of endometrial resection and ablation was 2.7/10,000.

Complications of hysterectomy

The complications of hysterectomy are often underestimated. Minor pyrexial morbidity was found in 47% of women after abdominal hysterectomy in the Pinion study with 11% having a vaginal vault haematoma and 5% requiring a blood transfusion.[10] There were also three major complications in that series.

The VALUE study in England and Wales is the largest and most recent assessment of complications.[16] This study reported 37,298 hysterectomies carried out for benign reasons in England and Wales during 1994 and 1995. Unlike the hysteroscopic surgery audits, unfortunately only 45% of hysterectomies during this period were reported. As the study in its ascertainment exercise found an under-reporting of major haemorrhage and return-to-theatre, the true figure may be higher than the study results suggest.

The mortality in this large series was 3.8/10,000. After abdominal hysterectomy for DUB the mortality was 2.5/10,000, virtually identical to that found in the ablation audits (2.7/10,000). The main causes of death were pulmonary embolus and heart disease. Overall, visceral damage occurred in 0.73%, major operative haemorrhage in 2.2%, and return-to-theatre in 0.75%. The total operative complication rate was 3.5%. Postoperative complications occurred in 8.5% of cases with a 1.0% rate of severe complications. Laparoscopic methods had the highest rates of operative complications and postoperative complications. Vaginal hysterectomy had a statistically significant lower rate of operative complications (odds ratio, 0.85; 95% CI, 0.74–0.97), but as the rate is similar (3.0% compared to 3.5%) the clinical significance is less clear. More postoperative complications occurred after vaginal than abdominal hysterectomy, 9.3% compared to 8.3% (95% CI, 1.05–1.22). The women in the vaginal group were older than in the abdominal group which may explain this small difference.[16].

In the US, 1851 premenopausal women undergoing hysterectomy were studied.[17] The hysterectomy was abdominal in 1283 and vaginal in 568 women. Pyrexia occurred after abdominal hysterectomy in 30%, and 15% needed a blood transfusion. Vaginal hysterectomy was followed by a pyrexia in 15%. Bowel injury occurred in 3/1000 women following abdominal hysterectomy and 6/1000 after vaginal hysterectomy. The urinary tract was damaged in 3/1000 after abdominal hysterectomy and in 14/1000 with vaginal hysterectomy

PATIENT SELECTION FOR ENDOMETRIAL ABLATION

Whilst some selection criteria are fairly obvious, others have become clearer as the evidence has accrued. From the beginning, the ablative procedures have only been offered to women whose family is complete because of probable sub-fertility and the potential risks to both to mother and fetus of a pregnancy following endometrial ablation. Since pregnancies could occur after ablation, women had to continue adequate contraception after the procedure. Ablation would not deal with a very large fibroid uterus.

There is now evidence as to the prognostic factors for successful ablation based on randomised trials and the large audit studies. Women whose menstrual blood loss is genuinely excessive have a better outcome after TCRE than those with normal menstrual blood loss. Gannon showed that, if menstrual blood loss was above 80 ml per cycle, the subjective failure rate was 9% compared to 18% if periods were perceived to be heavy but menstrual loss was normal.[18] Patient age may be important with younger women having a lower satisfaction than older women. The Scottish audit showed a lower satisfaction in women under 40 years of age, though this was still 79% as compared to 88% in women aged over 40 years.[13]

The presence of irregular periods or menstrual dysmenorrhoea is not a predictor of a poor outcome. In the trial comparing TCRE and ELA, there was no difference in satisfaction using each of these criteria.[15]

Whether endometrial ablation of the endometrium succeeds or fails is probably dependent on a number of variables, with genuine and perceived severity of symptoms, patient expectation and uterine pathology all playing their part. In addition, there is the individual variation in performance of the procedure. One method of determining reasons for the failure of endometrial ablation is to study the uterus in women after hysterectomy for failure. Though this tells nothing about the uterus in those women who have had a successful ablation.

Davis et al. have studied the histopathological status of the removed uterus following hysterectomy for failure of REA to control symptoms.[19] In women still complaining of bleeding excessively, they found that endometrium was present focally, but not diffusely, in the uterine cavity. Fibroids were found in 30% and adenomyosis in 27%. As already stated in the Pinion study, where the women had a clinical diagnosis of dysfunctional uterine bleeding, those randomised to hysterectomy were found to have endometriosis in 8%, adenomyosis in 17% and fibroids in 20%.[8] As the study was randomised, the same uterine pathology would be present in those women undergoing TCRE or ELA. Despite this, the hysterectomy rate 4–6 years after treatment is only 22%. It is probable that, in women with this range of pathology, many will have a satisfactory result from endometrial ablation if the indication for endometrial ablation is DUB rather than pain. Despite this knowledge, we still cannot reliably predict for an individual woman the outcome following endometrial ablation.

WHICH METHOD OF ENDOMETRIAL ABLATION?

A large number uncontrolled series of TCRE and ELA have been published as well as randomised studies comparing them to each other and to medical treatment. The two uncontrolled studies that give the best estimate as to the long-term outcome are the long-term follow-up studies of TCRE and ELA. Magos followed up 525 women for up to 5 years, though the mean follow-up was actually 31 months and only 43 women were followed up for the full 5 years. The hysterectomy rate was 9% and 80% avoided further surgery.[20] The Middlesborough group have reported long-term follow-up of 1000 ELA procedures, with 746 women followed up for up to 6 years. The rate of repeat surgery was 15% and, by using life table analysis, they predicted a hysterectomy rate of 21% at 6.5 years.[21] Despite the size of these studies, they are less useful than the long-term follow-up of RCTs. These studies, along with long-term follow-up of the Aberdeen randomised trial, show that the great majority of women will avoid a hysterectomy following first-generation endometrial ablation.

TCRE has been compared to ELA in a randomised trial of 372 patients.[15] This study showed that TCRE had a shorter operating time than ELA. Mean fluid absorption was less following TCRE and fewer patients absorbed a large volume during TCRE than with ELA. There were no differences in complications between the two methods and no difference in outcome as measured by satisfaction (90%), amenorrhoea rate (45%), or hysterectomy rate (20%).[15]

REA is a widely used method especially outside the UK, but has never been subject to a published randomised trial compared to hysterectomy or TCRE. Uncontrolled results give this method a similar success rate to the other hysteroscopic methods.

Second-generation ablative techniques represent a rapidly expanding area of medical technology. The majority use tissue heating as the method of endometrial destruction using electrical energy (Vesta system), microwave energy (Microwave Endometrial Ablation, MEA), laser (ELITT) or heated saline/glycine irrigating the uterus (Hydrotherm Ablator and circulating hot saline) or heated saline/dextrose contained within a balloon device (Thermachoice and Cavatherm systems). Second-generation techniques are mostly blind in nature (no hysteroscopy), most avoid the need for fluid distension media and its risks. They are quicker and much simpler to learn and perform than first-generation techniques, which many gynaecologists failed to master. Some also offer the benefits of local anaesthesia (MEA and Thermachoice).

These new procedures all post-date the earlier national safety audits.[13,14] The new techniques must prove equal efficacy but also safety before they can become widely accepted. Their efficacy should be compared in randomised trials of adequate power to the established gold standard of TCRE. Adequate training is vital to reduce the potential for serious complications with the second-generation techniques.

To date, the only methods which have been subject to adequate assessment are Thermachoice, MEA and the Vesta system. Thermal balloon has been compared in a RCT to REA. A multicentre North American trial randomised 275 women to thermal uterine balloon therapy (Thermachoice) or REA to study efficacy and safety.[22] The study was powered to detect 20% less efficacy for REA *versus* balloon. The study was restricted to women with small, regular uterine cavities and with high PBLAC scores. No pretreatment endometrial hormonal preparation was used and the endometrium was prepared with a 5-min suction aspiration. At 1 year, both techniques significantly reduced the PBLAC score, 68.4% in the REA arm and 61.6% in the balloon arm had a reduction of over 90% with no significant difference in the two groups. Quality-of-life scores, satisfaction and improvement in dysmenorrhoea/PMS were also similar. The balloon treatment was significantly quicker with no complications, compared to 3.2% of the REA group. The amenorrhoea rate was significantly lower after Thermachoice (15%) compared to (27%) after REA, despite the fact the amenorrhoea rate after REA was considerably less than expected with a first-generation method. This study was re-analysed at 2 and 3 years of follow-up.[23] At 2 years follow-up, 15 hysterectomies had been performed – 11 in the REA arm and 4 in the balloon arm. Of the 214 who were followed for 3 years, the results of uterine balloon therapy and REA remained similar, with little difference at 3 years compared with results at 1 year. The increase in hysterectomies in the REA group (14) compared with the uterine balloon therapy group (8) was not significant at 3 years.[23]

Both methods were considered highly successful at avoiding hysterectomy and relieving symptoms and patient satisfaction remained high.

Microwave Endometrial Ablation (MEA) has been validated against the gold standard of TCRE in a RCT. The procedure is blind, but many centres advocate routine carbon dioxide hysteroscopy following dilation to exclude perforation and false passages. The probe is 8 mm in diameter and delivers microwaves of 9.2 Ghz frequency to the probe tip. The Aberdeen group randomised 263 women to MEA or TCRE (the study had sufficient power to detect a 15% difference in satisfaction between the groups).[24] The inclusion criteria were the same as the previous studies,[3,10,15] specifically the uterus could to be up to the size of a 10 week pregnancy and fibroids were not excluded. MEA was a significantly faster procedure (11 *versus* 15 min) and had less operative complications. In the 2 year follow-up, 95% of the subjects returned questionnaires.[25] Similar menstrual data were reported in both arms with a higher amenorrhoea rate after MEA (47%) than TCRE (41%), which was not significant. Satisfaction was significantly higher after MEA with 79% of women either completely or generally satisfied compared to 67% after TCRE. Quality-of-life was similarly increased in both groups. Hysterectomy rates of 12% at 2 years were similar after both treatments. The group concluded that MEA was as effective as the TCRE.

A RCT comparing MEA under local anaesthetic (LA) compared to general anaesthetic (GA) is in press.[26] In this study of 359 women referred for MEA, 191 (59% of those eligible) agreed to randomisation to GA or LA and 131 (41%) agreed to participate in the patient preference arm of the study. Of the procedures started under LA, 91% were completed and 87% found LA totally or generally acceptable. Despite this, only 75% of those randomised to LA would have their treatment the same way, significantly less than those randomised to GA (88%).

The safety of MEA has been reported in a prospective series of 1400 cases.[27] The data covered 13 gynaecological units in the UK and Canada. Out of 1433 cases, one major complication of small bowel damage occurred giving an incidence of 7/10,000. There were few minor complications. In conclusion, MEA appeared safer than hysteroscopic methods.

The Vesta system – a disposable, dispensable multi-electrode carrying balloon utilising monopolar diathermy – has been compared in an RCT to combined resection/coagulation technique. Women who had menorrhagia as defined by PBLAC scoring (> 150) who had failed medical treatment with normal uterine cavities were randomised.[28] Out of the 557 women assessed as menorrhagic, only 244 were randomised, as approximately half proved unsuitable for the procedure by the other inclusion criteria. PBLACs were used in selection and definition of outcome success (a PBLAC score < 75 defined success). Success was achieved in 86.9% of the Vesta arm and 83% in TCRE at 1 year. Amenorrhoea rates were 31% in the Vesta arm and 34% in the TCRE arm. No significant complications were reported. With the Vesta procedures, 87% were performed under local anaesthesia ± sedation as an out-patient. Of note, there were 18 (10.6%) technical failures in the Vesta arm and one Vesta procedure had to be abandoned as the device had entered a weakened Caesarean scar. The benefits are avoiding fluid overload and local anaesthesia. The authors concluded that the Vesta method was equally effective and safe as TCRE. The Vesta system is, however, not currently marketed.

Hydrotherm Ablator, unlike the rest of the second-generation techniques, requires hysteroscopy. However, no manipulation by the operator is required. The technique relies upon circulating heated saline within the endometrial cavity. The saline is heated externally prior to being introduced into the hysteroscope and achieves an intra-uterine temperature of 90°C. This technique seems suitable for irregular cavities unlike the balloon methods. The device is 8 mm and takes 10 min of active treatment.

A multicentre RCT study comparing Hydrotherm Ablator (HTA) to REA has been published;[29] 276 patients with menorrhagia were randomised to HTA (187) or REA (89). PBLAC diaries were used for inclusion criteria and follow-up. Success was defined as a PBLAC score of < 75. Success rates as defined were 77% after HTA and 82% for REA. At one year, amenorrhoea rates were 40% with HTA and 51% with REA. The conclusion was that HTA was safe and effective, offered safety benefits with the associated use of hysteroscopy, and had the potential to be performed as an out-patient procedure.

With the exception of the trials on MEA, all the above trials on second-generation methods were initiated to obtain FDA approval in the US and were under the control of the device manufacturers.

Other techniques exist such as photodynamic therapy, cryo-ablation, circulating hot saline and Novacept. None of these have enough data to draw any conclusions. The ELITT device utilises an intra-uterine diode laser that scatters a laser beam around the endometrial cavity. Hysteroscopy is not required. The procedure is non-contact and claims to treat irregular cavities and areas difficult to access (*e.g.* the cornua). To date, evidence is limited to observational studies. Currently, the most thoroughly evaluated second-generation technique remains MEA.

CONCLUSIONS

Sufficient evidence is now available about the efficacy and safety of both hysterectomy and endometrial ablation. All patients with DUB will not want or be suitable for endometrial ablation, but should be correctly counselled and offered endometrial ablation as well as hysterectomy. As results and safety are broadly similar, the recovery time, possible avoidance of a general anaesthetic and especially patient choice are the important factors.

The second-generation methods must be assessed rigorously, similar to the first-generation methods. Those that prove efficacious and safe will allow endometrial ablation to be provided by the majority of gynaecologists.

Key points for clinical practice

- Women must be offered a choice of surgical treatments for dysfunctional uterine bleeding after accurate non-directional counselling.

- Both hysterectomy and endometrial ablation offer similar satisfaction for the treatment of dysfunctional uterine bleeding.

- Endometrial ablation should not be withheld in a woman who does not wish to try medical treatment.

- The rate of bowel and urinary tract damage appears to be similar following both endometrial ablation and hysterectomy, but there are fewer major complications and recovery is much faster with endometrial ablation.

- The majority (80%) of women will avoid hysterectomy after a first-generation method of endometrial ablation. The satisfaction rate is around 85% with 35–40% achieving amenorrhoea.

- The second-generation methods of endometrial ablation must be rigorously assessed. Microwave endometrial ablation and Thermachoice have achieved this. Amenorrhoea is found in 15% of women after Thermachoice and > 40% after microwave endometrial ablation.

References

1. Reid PC, Cocker A, Coltart R. Assessment of menstrual blood loss using a pictorial chart: a validation study. *Br J Obstet Gynaecol* 2000; **107**: 320–322
2. Parkin DE. Prognostic factors for endometrial ablation and resection. *Lancet* 1998; **351**: 1147–1148.
3. Cooper KG, Parkin DE, Garret AM, Grant AM. Two year follow-up of women randomised to medical management or transcervical resection of the endometrium for heavy menstrual loss; clinical and quality of life outcomes. *Br J Obstet Gynaecol* 1999; **106**: 258–265.
4. Cooper KG, Jack SA, Parkin DE, Grant AM. Five-year follow up of women randomised to medical management or transcervical resection of the endometrium for heavy menstrual loss: clinical and quality of life outcomes. *Br J Obstet Gynaecol* 2001; **108**: 1222–1228.
5. Crosignani PG, Vercellini P, Mosconi P *et al*. Levonorgestrel-releasing intrauterine device *versus* hysteroscopic endometrial resection in the treatment of dysfunctional uterine bleeding. *Obstet Gynecol* 1997; **90**: 257–263.
6. Lahteenmaki P, Haukkamaa M, Puolakka J *et al*. Open randomised study of use of levonorgestrel releasing intrauterine system as alternative to hysterectomy. *BMJ* 1998; **316**: 1122–1126.
7. Hurskainen R, Teperi J, Rissanen P *et al*. Quality of life and cost-effectiveness of levonorgestrel-releasing intrauterine system versus hysterectomy for treatment of menorrhagia: a randomised trial. *Lancet* 2001; **357**: 273–277.
8. Gannon MJ, Holt EM, Fairbank J *et al*. A randomised trial comparing endometrial resection and abdominal hysterectomy for the treatment of menorrhagia. *BMJ* 1991; **303**: 1362–1364.
9. Dwyer N, Hutton J, Stirrat GM. Randomised controlled trial comparing endometrial resection with abdominal hysterectomy for the surgical treatment of menorrhagia. *Br J Obstet Gynaecol* 1993; **100**: 237–243.
10. Pinion SB, Parkin DE, Abramovich DR *et al*. Randomised trial of hysterectomy, endometrial laser ablation and transcervical resection for dysfunctional uterine bleeding. *BMJ* 1994; **309**: 979–983.
11. Aberdeen Endometrial Ablation Trials Group. A randomised trial of endometrial ablation versus hysterectomy for the treatment of dysfunctional uterine bleeding: outcome at four years. *Br J Obstet Gynaecol* 1999; **106**: 360–366.
12. O'Connor H, Broadbent J, Magos A, McPherson K. Medical Research Council randomised trial of endometrial resection *versus* hysterectomy in the management of menorrhagia. *Lancet* 1997; **349**: 891–901.
13. Scottish Hysteroscopy Audit Group. A Scottish audit of hysteroscopic surgery for menorrhagia: complications and follow up. *Br J Obstet Gynaecol* 1995; **102**: 249–254.
14. Overton C, Hargreaves H, Maresh M. A national survey of the complications of endometrial destruction for menstrual disorders: the MISTLETOE study. *Br J Obstet Gynaecol* 1997; **104**: 1351–1359.
15. Bhattacharya S, Cameron IM, Parkin DE *et al*. A pragmatic randomised comparison of transcervical resection of the endometrium with endometrial laser ablation for the treatment of menorrhagia. *Br J Obstet Gynaecol* 1997; **104**: 601–607.
16. Maresh MJA, Metcalfe MA, McPherson K *et al*. The VALUE national hysterectomy study: description of the patients and their surgery. *Br J Obstet Gynaecol* 2002; **109**: 302–312.
17. Dicker RC, Greenspan JR, Strauss LT. Complications of abdominal and vaginal hysterectomy among women of reproductive age in the United States. *Am J Obstet Gynecol* 1982; **144**: 841–848.
18. Gannon MJ, Day P, Hammadich N, Johnston N. A new method of measuring menstrual blood loss and its use in screening women before endometrial ablation. *Br J Obstet Gynaecol* 1996; **103**: 1029–1033.
19. Davis JR, Maynard KK, Brainard CP *et al*. Effects of thermal endometrial ablation: clinicopathologic correlations. *Am J Clin Pathol* 1998; **109**: 96–100.
20. O'Connor H, Magos A. Endometrial resection for the treatment of menorrhagia. *N Engl J Med* 1996; **335**: 151–156.

21. Phillips G, Chien PF, Garry R. Risk of hysterectomy after 1000 consecutive endometrial laser ablations. *Br J Obstet Gynaecol* 1998; **105**: 897–903.
22. Mayer WR, Walsh BW, Grainger JF *et al*. Thermal balloon and rollerball ablation to treat menorrhagia: a multicenter comparison. *Obstet Gynecol* 1998; **92**: 98–103.
23. Loffer FD. Three-year comparison of thermal balloon and rollerball ablation in treatment of menorrhagia. *J Am Assoc Gynecol Laparosc* 2001; **81**: 48–54.
24. Cooper KG, Bain C, Parkin DE. Comparison of microwave endometrial ablation and transcervical resection of the endometrium for treatment of heavy menstrual loss: a randomised trial. *Lancet* 1999; **354**: 1859–1863.
25. Bain C, Cooper KG, Parkin DE. Microwave endometrial ablation *versus* endometrial resection: a randomised controlled trial. *Obstet Gynecol* 2002; **99**: 983–987.
26. Wallage S, Cooper KG, Graham W, Parkin DE. A prospective randomised controlled trial comparing microwave endometrial ablation under local and general anaesthetic, acceptability and clinical outcome. *Br J Obstet Gynaecol* 2003; In press.
27. Parkin DE. Microwave endometrial ablation: a safe technique. Complication data from a prospective series of 1400 cases. *Gynaecol Endosc* 2000; **9**: 385–388.
28. Corson SL, Brill AI, Brooks PG *et al*. One-year results of the Vesta system for endometrial ablation. *J Am Assoc Gynecol Laparosc* 2000; **7**: 489–497.
29. Corson SL. A multicenter evaluation of endometrial ablation by Hydrotherm Ablator and rollerball for treatment of menorrhagia. *J Am Assoc Gynecol Laparosc* 2001; **8**: 359–367.

John Reidy Bruce McLucas

11

Evaluation of arterial embolisation of uterine fibroids

Although uterine artery embolisation (UAE) is a relatively new technique, percutaneous trans-catheter embolisation has been practised by radiologists for well over 20 years. In many different clinical situations, a great variety of embolisation materials or agents has been used in various parts of the body, but generally these procedures are only occasionally performed. One important indication is severe bleeding not responding to conservative measures, where the alternative treatment would involve major surgery. Embolisation has also been used in tumours, particularly where they are hypervascular, when the role has often been to debulk and devascularise immediately prior to surgery. The third main indication is in arteriovenous malformations and fistulae. In 1995, UAE was first advocated as a treatment for uterine fibroids.[1]

First described in 1979, embolisation of the uterus has been reported in a variety of conditions including postpartum haemorrhage and bleeding following Caesarean section or gynaecological surgery, haemorrhage after ectopic pregnancy, arteriovenous malformations and in gynaecological cancer.[2-4] In 1995, Ravina, a gynaecologist in Paris, described embolisation as a pre-operative adjunct to surgery in 31 patients.[1] One year later, the same group reported on 16 patients in whom UAE was used as the primary treatment.[5] They selectively catheterised both uterine arteries, which were then embolised with polyvinyl alcohol particles to the point of complete occlusion. At a mean follow-up of 20 months, 11 patients had a good clinical result, with 3 partial improvements and only 2 failures that progressed to surgery. Since this report, there has been great interest in this procedure, particularly from interventional radiologists. The literature on this procedure is not large and, though good long-term data are still not available, it is being increasingly accepted with an estimated 20,000 women having been treated.

John Reidy FRCR FRCP, Consultant Vascular and Interventional Radiologist, Guy's and St Thomas' Hospital, St Thomas Street, London SE1 9RT, UK (for correspondence)

Bruce McLucas MD, Department of Obstetrics and Gynaecology, 100 UCLA Medical Plaza, Suite 310, Los Angeles, CA 90024, USA. E-mail: mclucas@ucla.edu

INDICATIONS

Embolisation is only advocated for fibroids associated with significant symptoms. The indications for UAE for uterine fibroids are the same as for hysterectomy or myomectomy. One important difference between UAE and surgical procedures is that pathological confirmation of uterine fibroid disease is not obtained in UAE and the spectre is always raised that a uterine sarcoma could be missed.[6,7] Uterine sarcomas are, however, extremely rare and their clinical presentation is usually different. If there is any suggestion that a sarcoma could be present, particularly in older women, then further investigation with magnetic resonance imaging (MRI) is indicated.[8] Adenomyosis may present with symptoms similar to uterine fibroids and, being relatively common, the two conditions may co-exist. Though embolisation has been advocated for adenomyosis, no data suggest that embolisation is effective in this condition.

For a variety of reasons, many women choose not to undergo, or are reluctant to submit to, a hysterectomy. This is particularly so in Afro-Caribbean women. In addition to seeking a uterus-conserving treatment, the morbidity of surgery and the time lost from work following surgery has led many women to seek less invasive options. Myomectomy as a surgical alternative may not be suitable for certain patients and involves the risk of severe bleeding and hysterectomy. Thus, many women will self-select for UAE as there is wide-spread awareness of the procedure from publicity and information carried on the internet. Many women approach their gynaecologist with a fair degree of knowledge about fibroid embolisation.

CONTRA-INDICATIONS

At present, all types of fibroid disease are considered suitable for UAE with the exception of pedunculated subserous fibroids. Cases have been reported where necrotic subserous fibroids have resulted in bowel adhesions and the need for laparotomy. The other contra-indication to the procedure is the presence of pelvic inflammatory disease, which should be excluded clinically. Women who would not consider a hysterectomy in any circumstances should also not be considered.

It is not uncommon for fibroids which are asymptomatic to be noted on routine ultrasound or computed tomography. These women need to be reassured that no treatment is necessary.

IMAGING AND ASSESSMENT PRIOR TO THE EMBOLISATION

All patients should be assessed by a gynaecologist to confirm the clinical diagnosis and to determine whether the fibroids are the cause of significant symptoms. Women should be assessed prior to UAE, and followed up by the same gynaecologist who can be readily consulted in the event of any possible complications.[9]

In addition to a recent gynaecological assessment, some form of routine imaging, usually ultrasound, is advised. MRI will demonstrate fibroids in much greater detail, but the cost considerations will often restrict its use.[8]

It is important to exclude the presence of any pelvic inflammatory disease that would be a contra-indication to UAE. A cervical swab may be taken, but our approach is to exclude infection by the clinical history and examination. A pregnancy test should be routinely performed.[9]

One of the concerns following UAE is amenorrhoea which has rarely been reported but particularly important in younger women. It is advisable to obtain follicle-stimulating hormone (FSH) levels on all women under the age of 45 years on day 3 of their cycle as this will give a pointer to a possible early menopause.

EMBOLISATION TECHNIQUE

Before consenting to UAE, all women must be given a clear account of the realistic expectations of the procedure with an explanation of exactly what embolisation entails. This is best achieved with a patient information leaflet.[9] The radiologist must be available to deal with any questions or concerns. It is particularly important to explain that severe pain usually results immediately following the procedure and to detail how this will be effectively managed. In the United States, UAE is performed as a day-case procedure in some centres but we advise an overnight admission because of the pain felt after the procedure and the post-embolisation syndrome. Radiologists should only attempt these procedures when they are well experienced with arteriography and embolisation techniques. The procedures should be carried out using state-of-the-art angiographic equipment that will enable the X-ray dose to be kept to a minimum.

The technique, using a standard arteriographic approach, involves selectively catheterising both uterine arteries and embolising them to the point of complete or near-total occlusion. No attempt is made to catheterise and embolise selectively the fibroids as opposed to the remainder of the uterus. Some have advocated a co-axial embolisation (double-catheter) technique, but this increases the complexity of the procedure, the time taken, the radiation dose, and also increases the cost.[10,11] Other radiologists have found it difficult to catheterise both uterine arteries from the one femoral artery approach and prefer a bilateral femoral arterial access.[12] The aim is to position the tip of the catheter safely into both uterine arteries; filming is only necessary to confirm this and to demonstrate the vascularity of the uterine artery and the fibroid uterus. The uterine arteries have a characteristically tortuous course, are normally fairly low in the pelvis, and usually course medially and anteriorly. Usually a small (4-F) catheter and steerable guide wire combination are used by the experienced angiographer. However, the procedure can sometimes prove difficult and technical failure occurs rarely.

The uterus is supplied by paired uterine arteries and, with rare exceptions, no other arteries need to be considered; they are usually of equal size, but there may be some asymmetry.[13,14] Abnormal vessels surround the fibroid with a corkscrew-like appearance and marked vascularity – often the shape of fibroids is outlined by the abnormal vascularity. The aim of the embolisation is to occlude the vascular bed and the main artery to the point of near total occlusion. This is achieved by injecting particulate emboli mixed with contrast medium until the forward flow in the artery has been abolished and there is a tendency to reflux into the main internal iliac artery. Polyvinyl alcohol (PVA) particles, which have been used in embolisation for over 20 years, are most commonly used.[15] These come in a range of particle sizes and 500 µm particles aremost often used. Quite large quantities may be needed to effect occlusion in a large fibroid uterus and the PVA particles are often supplemented by the injection of a suspension of Gelfoam. Gelfoam, which is much less expensive than PVA, may achieve the same result but is biodegradable and the particle size is less controllable.

Though PVA is well established as a particulate embolisation agent, the sized particles can be quite irregular in shape with a tendency to clump in suspension resulting in an embolisation procedure that is not uniform. Embosphere microspheres are microbeads specifically designed for embolisation and have been advocated particularly for UAE.[16] It is suggested that they give a more uniform embolisation with less post-embolisation syndrome, but no good data support this.

There is a real concern about UAE, particularly in younger women, as the ovaries are directly in the X-ray beam for much of the examination.[17] Every possible measure should be used to decrease the amount of radiation. State-of-the-art angiographic equipment with dose-reduction features including pulsed fluoroscopy are important. The skill of the angiographer should enable fluoroscopy times to be kept to a reasonable level. Limited filming is only necessary to demonstrate selective catheterisation of the uterine artery. If attention to these measures is not given, high X-ray doses can result which are equivalent to several barium enema studies.[10] This is particularly important in younger women who may possibly want to become pregnant.

Prior to starting up a UAE programme, a pain-relief protocol should be established and anaesthetists and pain-relief specialists consulted. Women should be monitored throughout the procedure. The approach at Guy's & St Thomas' Hospital is to give intravenous sedation at the beginning of the procedure. Pain does not occur until the second uterine artery is embolised and it is important to give strong analgesics just prior to this stage. We give an intramuscular injection of 10 mg morphine and, at the end of the procedure, we establish an intravenous patient-controlled analgesia (PCA) pump set to give 1-mg boluses of morphine with 6-min lock-out periods. We find that non-steroidal anti-inflammatory drugs such as Diclofenac 100 mg given as a suppository either alone or combined with the PCA are effective following the procedure and can be repeated once after 12 h. The post-embolisation syndrome, as well as the morphine, is likely to result in some nausea and vomiting and it is important to prescribe anti-emetics. With rare exceptions, women are able to go home the next day, but a supply of analgesics are given as some less severe pain may persist for 2–3 weeks. Patients are advised to take about 2 weeks off work, but some are able to go back to work sooner.

There are real concerns regarding the risk of infection following UAE and this can occur several months later with necrotic fibroids. Many radiologists will routinely give prophylactic antibiotics at the time of the procedure even though there are no good data to support this approach. Based on the gynaecological surgical experience and the knowledge that anaerobic infections may occur, giving a single dose of metronidazole with a cephalosporin or quinalone drug has been recommended.[9]

RESULTS

Limited and less than satisfactory data are available on the results following UAE. No randomised controlled data are as yet available and there are no long-term results. In the limited literature of about 1000 women, a variety of methods have been used to assess the clinical results, all of them short-term evaluations.[18–22]

Furthermore, these assessments are made more difficult as it seems to be generally accepted that these are difficult women to assess and many of them present with high expectations of this uterus-conserving procedure. Notwithstanding the limitations of these assessments, the overall results suggest that 80–90% of the patients are happy with their clinical result. In addition to the symptomatic assessment of patients, objective assessments have been made of the degree of fibroid shrinkage and overall uterine size reduction. Both ultrasound and MRI evaluations have been used, with MRI being the more sensitive and precise technique for measurement.[8,23] An overall fibroid size reduction of around 50% has been reported, which may take up to 6 months and more before it is complete.

After the initial enthusiasm for UAE, many workers are now establishing better health-related quality-of-life assessment protocols and,[24–26] in a number of countries, registries are being established which should allow better data to be obtained. Ideally, a randomised controlled study should be established with UAE compared with surgery. Despite general acceptance of this methodology, real concerns exist that recruitment of women to such a trial will prove difficult.

COMPLICATIONS

POST-EMBOLISATION SYNDROME

The post-embolisation syndrome, of which pain is the most important feature, occurs in a majority of women following UAE. Nausea and vomiting and a feeling of general malaise are also features of this syndrome which may last for up to 2 weeks. Potentially, local femoral artery complications can occur as with any arteriography procedure, but the use of small catheters in non-atheromatous patients makes this very unlikely. Some moderate haematoma can occur following any arteriographic procedure. Contrast reactions are now extremely rare. There is a possibility that other arteries can be embolised (non-target embolisation), but this should be wholly preventable by good embolisation technique and careful fluoroscopy during the embolisation procedure. Reflux from the uterine artery would embolise other branches of the internal iliac and, unless significant reflux occurred, this would have no clinical sequelae. Our experience suggests that technical failure occurs in about 2.5% of patients due to an inability to achieve selective catheterisation of a very tortuous uterine artery. Anomalies rarely occur with a small or non-existent uterine artery on one side.

Some discharge is quite common, starting a few days after the procedure and lasting several weeks. This is usually an intermittent, non-purulent discharge and sometimes fragments of fibroids may be passed. If the discharge becomes offensive or is associated with pain or fever, infection should be suspected and the patient urgently assessed with a view to treatment.

LATE COMPLICATIONS

The early experience of UAE did not pay much attention to complications. Serious complications, though rare, do occur. Two deaths have been reported following UAE. In one, a woman re-presented 11 days post-uterine artery embolisation with septic shock. Blood cultures grew *Escherichia coli* and, despite a hysterectomy, she never recovered. The second case was reported from Italy with only limited data available, where a 60-year-old woman known to have breast cancer died of a massive pulmonary embolism one day following the procedure.

Hysterectomy is a significant complication especially as most women choose UAE as a result of a strong desire to avoid the operation. Hysterectomy may be carried out when there has been no clinical response and very rarely for severe pain. The most common cause for hysterectomy is infection associated with necrotic fibroids. This is more common in women with large fibroids and the overall incidence is of the order of 1%. It is important that, before consenting to UAE, all women are notified of this hysterectomy risk. This post-UAE hysterectomy may present up to 3–4 months later and the operation can prove to be difficult because of bowel adhesions. Infection occurs more commonly in association with chronic vaginal discharge. If there is any suggestion of infection, women should seek medical attention early for diagnosis and treatment with antibiotics. Sometimes, ancillary gynaecological procedures such as suction evacuation or fibroid removal are necessary. Hopefully, this awareness of infection and the associated risks will keep the incidence of hysterectomy at a minimum.

Fibroid expulsion or sloughing of fibroids occurs in 3–8% of cases and is particularly common in submucous fibroids. It is important to explain to women prior to the procedure that this may occur as it can cause considerable alarm to both patient and gynaecologist especially when a large fibroid is passed. Expulsion can be associated with significant pain and haemorrhage and may need some gynaecological intervention. Generally, when fibroids are passed vaginally, this is associated with a good clinical outcome.

Cervical fibroids present as a particular problem when they are not accessible to a hysteroscopic approach. Myomectomy via an abdominal approach is then associated with a significant risk of hysterectomy. These cases would appear to respond well to UAE with the likelihood that the fibroid will shrink and subsequently be passed vaginally. Such patients need very careful follow-up as they will usually require a gynaecological procedure.

The other serious complication following UAE is amenorrhoea and premature menopause especially when this occurs in younger women. Amenorrhoea has been reported in up to 5% of women following UAE, but many of these cases are in women over the age of 45 years or when the amenorrhoea was temporary. Probably, true ovarian failure in younger women is rare and of the order of less than 1%; however, again it is important to counsel women that this is a rare, but possible, complication.

FIBROIDS AND FERTILITY

Though fibroids are commonly associated with infertility and miscarriages, embolisation is not currently recommended unless the fibroids are also associated with significant symptoms. There are innate concerns regarding UAE in women who may want to become pregnant in the future. Some have suggested that it should not be used in such women due to the lack of research into the long-term effects of UAE on both fertility and the child. However, this must be balanced against the view that there are no easy choices for infertile women with large fibroids. The reality is that there are only two reasonable uterus conserving options – myomectomy and embolisation. The data for fertility following myomectomy are better than after UAE. A number of papers attest to normal pregnancies following embolisation as experience of this procedure increases.[28-31] In a recent paper, 139 women out of 400 who underwent UAE stated a desire for fertility after the embolisation. Of these, only 52 were under the age of 40 years and their progress was closely followed; 17 pregnancies occurred in 14 women. The course of their pregnancies and their deliveries were unremarkable suggesting that the risk compared favourably with that of patients undergoing myomectomy.[32] In younger women who are concerned about future fertility, myomectomy should be weighed against UAE. Factors affecting the choice include gynaecological experience of myomectomy, number and size of fibroids, and the woman's own preferences having been given all the available information.

Key points for clinical practice

- Uterine artery embolisation is a relatively new technique which may be applicable to the majority of women with fibroids.

- Early results are encouraging with the majority of the women being satisfied with the procedure and the low risk of complications.

- At present, the data are short-term and longer term controlled studies are required to establish the place of embolisation in the treatment of fibroids.

References

1. Ravina JH, Bouret JM, Fried D et al. Value of pre-operative embolisation of a uterine fibroma: report of a multi-centre series of 31 cases. Contracept Fertil Sex 1995; 23: 45–49.
2. Vedantham S, Goodwin SC, McLucas B, Mohr G. Uterine artery embolisation – an under-used method of controlling pelvic haemorrhage. Am J Obstet Gynecol 1999; 176: 938–948.
3. Greenwood LH, Glickman MG, Schwartz PE, Morse S, Denny DF. Obstetric and non-malignant gynecologic bleeding: treatment with angiographic embolization. Radiology 1987; 164: 155–159.
4. Abbas FM, Currie JL, Mitchell S et al. Selective vascular embolization in benign gynecologic conditions. J Reprod Med 1994; 39: 492–496.
5. Ravina JH, Herbreteau D, Ciraru-Vigneron N et al. Arterial embolisation to treat uterine myomata. Lancet 1995; 346: 671–672.
6. Parker WH, Fu YS, Berek JS. Uterine sarcoma in patients operated on for presumed leiomyoma and rapidly growing leiomyoma. Obstet Gynecol 1994; 83: 414–418.
7. Al-Badr A, Faught W. Uterine artery embolization in an undiagnosed uterine sarcoma. Obstet Gynecol 2001; 97: 836–837.

8. Jha RC, Ascher SM, Imaoka I, Spies JB. Symptomatic fibroleiomyoma: MR imaging of the uterus before and after uterine arterial embolization. *Radiology* 2000; **217**: 222–235.

9. Joint Working Party, Royal College of Radiologists and The Royal College of Obstetricians and Gynaecologists UK. *Clinical Recommendations on the Use of Uterine Artery Embolisation in the Management of Fibroids.* London: RCOG Press, 2000.

10. Nikolic B, Spies JB, Campbell L, Walsh SM, Abbara S, Lundsten MJ. Uterine artery embolization: reduced radiation with refined technique. *J Vasc Interv Radiol* 2001; **12**: 39–44.

11. Pelage JP, LeDref O, Soyer P *et al.* Fibroid-related menorrhagia: treatment with superselective embolization of the uterine arteries and mid-term follow-up. *Radiology* 2000; **215**: 428–431.

12. Pelage JP, Soyer P, Le Dref O *et al.* Uterine arteries: bilateral catheterisation with a single femoral approach and a single 5-F catheter. *Radiology* 1999; **210**: 573–575.

13. Pelage JP, Le Dref O, Soyer P *et al.* Arterial anatomy of the female genital tract: variations and relevance to transcatheter embolization of the uterus. *AJR Am J Roentgenol* 1998; **172**: 989–994.

14. Sampson JA. The blood supply of uterine myomata. *Surg Gynecol Obstet* 1912; **14**: 215–224.

15. Siskin GP, Englander M, Stainken BF, Ahn J, Dowling K, Dolen EG. Embolic agent used for uterine fibroid embolization. *AJR Am J Roentgenol* 2000; **175**: 767–773.

16. Spikes JB, Benenati JE, Worthington-Kirsch RL, Pelage JP. Initial experience with use of trisacryl gelatin microspheres for uterine artery embolization for leiomyomata. *J Vasc Interv Radiol* 2001; **12**: 1059–1063.

17. Nikolic B, Spies JB, Lundsten MJ, Abbara S. Patient radiation dose associated with uterine artery embolization. *Radiology* 2000; **214**: 121–125.

18. Worthington-Kirsch RL, Popky GL, Hutchins FL. Uterine arterial embolisation for the management of leiomyomas: quality of life assessment and clinical response. *Radiology* 1998; **208**: 652–659.

19. Bradley EA, Reidy JF, Forman RG, Jarosz J, Braude PR. Transcatheter uterine artery embolisation to treat large uterine fibroids. *Br J Obstet Gynaecol* 1998; **105**: 235–240.

20. Hutchins FL, Worthington-Kirsch RL, Berkowitz RP. Selective uterine artery embolization as primary treatment for symptomatic leiomyomata uteri: a review of 305 consecutive cases. *J Am Assoc Gynecol Laparosc* 1999; **6**: 279–284.

21. Spies JB, Scialli AR, Jha RC *et al.* Initial results from uterine fibroid embolization for symptomatic leiomyomata. *J Vasc Interv Radiol* 1999; **10**: 1159–1165.

22. McLucas B, Adler L, Perella R. Uterine fibroid embolization: nonsurgical treatment for symptomatic fibroids. *J Am Coll Surg* 2001; **192**: 95–105.

23. Burn P, McCall J, Chinn R, Vashisht A, Smith J, Healy J. Uterine fibroleiomyoma: MR imaging appearances before and after uterine arterial embolization. *Radiology* 2000; **217**: 222–235.

24. McLucas B, Adler L, Perrella R. Predictive factors for success in uterine fibroid embolization. *Minim Invasive Ther Allied Technol* 1999; **8**: 429–432.

25. Spies JB, Warren EH, Mathias SD, Walsh SM, Roth AR, Pentecost MJ. Uterine fibroid embolization: measurement of health-related quality-of-life before and after therapy. *J Vasc Interv Radiol* 1999; **10**: 1293–1303.

26. Subramanian S, Spies JB. Uterine artery embolization for leiomyomata: resource use and cost estimation. *J Vasc Interv Radiol* 2001; **21**: 571–574.

27. Vashisht A, Studd J, Carey A, Burn P. Fatal septicaemia after fibroid embolisation. *Lancet* 1999; **354**: 9175.

28. Nott V, Reidy JF, Forman RG, Braude P. Complications of fibroid embolization. *Minim Invasive Ther Allied Technol* 1999; **8**: 421–424.

29. Poppe W, Van Assche FA, Wilms G, Favril A, Baert A. Pregnancy after transcatheter embolization of a uterine arteriovenous malformation. *Am J Obstet Gynecol* 1987; **156**: 1179–1180.

30. Stancato-Pasik A, Mitty HA, Richard HM, Eshkar N. Obstetric embolotherapy: effect on menses and pregnancy. *Radiology* 1997; **204**: 791–793.

31. Ravina JH, Ciraru-Vigneron N, Aymard A, Le Dref O, Merland JJ. Pregnancy after embolization of uterine myoma: report of 12 cases. *Fertil Steril* 2000; **73**: 1241–1243.

32. Christmas HB, Saker MB, Ryu R *et al.* The impact of uterine fibroid embolization on resumption of menses and ovarian function. *J Vasc Interv Radiol* 2002; **11**: 699–703.

Fiona Reid Anthony R.B. Smith

12

Reducing the complications of minimal access pelvic surgery

In the last 20 years, the field of endoscopic surgery has expanded dramatically and now many gynaecological operations can be undertaken laparoscopically. The world literature contains many articles describing new techniques of performing almost every traditional operation endoscopically.

Endoscopic surgery does present new challenges. Additional training is required. There are inherent risks in many laparoscopic procedures, which may add to the risks of the basic procedure. The instrumentation is often more complex and may produce additional hazards.

The first principle of reducing complications is good training including coverage of the theory and practice of the surgical techniques involved. Many complications occur because this essential aspect has been overlooked or ignored.

AIMS OF ENDOSCOPIC SURGERY

An endoscopic approach to a surgical procedure aims to provide benefits to the patient, surgeon and health service provider. Patients should experience less pain, reduced peri-operative morbidity, less visible scarring, and a speedier return to normal function.

The surgeon should benefit from a better display of anatomy and pathology. There is also less exposure to the risk of infections such as hepatitis and HIV. Health care providers and society should benefit from reduced costs of in-patient care and the quicker return to normal function. Each new endoscopic procedure should be judged against these standards. At present, there is more opinion than evidence as to whether these standards are met.

Fiona Reid MB ChB MRCOG
Clinical Research Fellow, The Warrell Unit, St Mary's Hospital, Whitworth Park, Manchester M13 0JH, UK

Anthony R.B. Smith MB ChB FRCOG MD, Consultant Gynaecologist, The Warrell Unit, St Mary's Hospital, Whitworth Park, Manchester M13 0JH, UK (for correspondence)

OVERALL RISK OF LAPAROSCOPIC SURGERY

A recent meta-analysis[1] of 27 randomised control trials comparing laparoscopic procedures for benign gynaecological conditions with their equivalent open procedures found the overall risk of complications was significantly lower for patients undergoing the laparoscopic procedure (Relative risk, 0.59; 95% CI, 0.5–0.7) No statistically significant difference was found in the risk of major complications (relative risk, 1.0; 95% CI, 0.6–1.65).

However, although this was a meta-analysis of 27 trials, the actual number of women involved was small; only 3611 women were randomised. The analysis also combined a wide range of procedures from tubal ligation to hysterectomy.

Kreb[2] studied the incidence of bowel injury in all gynaecological surgery (Table 1) and found no evidence that laparoscopic surgery was more likely to cause injury to bowel than other methods of gynaecological surgery.

Table 1 Incidence of bowel injury in all gynaecological surgery[2]

Type of surgery	Number of cases	Total frequency of bowel injury	Frequency of entry-related bowel injury
Laparotomy	5700	16.3/1000	8.4/1000
Vaginal	985	11.4/1000	7.3/1000
Laparoscopic	3710	3.5/1000	3.0/1000

ANAESTHETIC RISKS

Over the last decade, there has been a change in both the type of laparoscopic operations performed and the population of patients undergoing surgery. In the past, short procedures were performed electively on young healthy women, for example laparoscopic sterilizations. Now, longer procedures, such as pelvic floor reconstruction, may be performed on an elderly population. Laparoscopic salpingectomies are performed, for ectopic pregnancies, on patients who may be hypovolaemic.

Most of the literature about cardiopulmonary function during laparoscopy is from studies on young healthy women undergoing elective procedures. The factors in laparoscopic surgery that affect anaesthetic parameters are raised intra-abdominal pressure, insufflation of CO_2, and the position of the patient. There are three main ventilatory problems that can occur during laparoscopy – increased $PaCO_2$, pneumothorax, and gas embolism. $PaCO_2$ increases more in patients with higher ASA.[3]

Gas can dissect through congenital abnormalities and can result in bilateral pneumothoracies.[4] Gas embolism is rare and occurs mainly during induction of pneumoperitoneum. Usually CO_2 gas embolism resolves rapidly, because CO_2 is very soluble in blood, but if it its large enough it can be fatal.

The Trendelenburg position does not have a significant effect on cardiopulmonary function in healthy individuals; however, there is currently insufficient evidence about the effects in patients with cardiopulmonary insufficiency, the obese or the elderly. The results of studies of cardiopulmonary function during

Table 2 Incidence of major bowel and major vascular injury following laparoscopic entry

Study	Number of cases	Bowel injury rate	Vascular injury rate
Mintz[6]	99,204	0.3/1000	0.5/1000
Loffer & Pent[7]	32,719	0.7/1000	Not recorded
Bergqvist & Bergqvist[8]	75,035	Not recorded	0.07/1000
Chapron et al.[9]	29,966	0.5/1000	0.2/1000
Harkki-Siren et al.[10]	102,812	0.3/1000	0.1/1000
Total	339,736	0.4/1000	0.2/1000

laparoscopic cholecystectomy may not be applicable to gynaecological procedures because cholecystectomy is performed in the reverse Trendelenburg position.

Pneumoperitoneum is associated with 25-35% drop in cardiac output. Raised intra-abdominal pressure is associated with reduced perfusion of abdominal organs. At 20 mmHg, intra-abdominal pressure, renal blood flow and glomerular filtration are 25% of normal and mesenteric blood flow is reduced;[4] however, the clinical significance of these changes is unknown. Small case series suggest that with expertise in anaesthetics and surgery, laparoscopy is safe even in high-risk patients.[5]

LAPAROSCOPIC ENTRY INJURIES

The incidence of major bowel injury during laparoscopic entry has been estimated from several large series at 1 in 2500 cases and major vascular injury at 1 in 5000 (Table 2).

Although the incidence of major complications is low, laparoscopy is a common procedure; over 123,000 laparoscopies are performed in the UK each year, and hence 75 women can be expected to sustain a severe complication each year.[11]

The injuries can have serious sequelae, including laparotomy, bowel resections, vascular grafts, and even death. In the context of a minor procedure, these are major complications and all surgeons should adopt a safe approach to laparoscopic entry. The method employed to gain access to the abdominal cavity remains one of the most debated topics among laparoscopists. Since the injury rates are low, the size of clinical trials required to demonstrate that one technique is safer than another is prohibitively large. In order to demonstrate a 50% reduction in bowel injury from 0.4/1000 to 0.2/1000 would require 260,000 cases in a randomised controlled trial.

This lack of evidence does not give surgeons *carte blanche* to use unrecognised methods of entry. There are consensus opinions about safe entry techniques[12] and surgeons who fail to employ recommended techniques may experience difficulty defending an adverse event in court.

MINIMISING VASCULAR INJURIES DURING LAPAROSCOPIC ENTRY

The reported incidence of vascular injuries varies possibly due to a lack of definition of a major vascular injury and a focus on the great vessels. The methods of data collection and observational study design may also affect the

Box 1 Risk factors for vascular damage

Failure to note anatomical landmarks
Position of the patient
Inadequate pneumoperitoneum
The depth of insertion of the Veress or trocar
Lateral deviation of the Veress or trocar
Perpendicular insertion of the Veress or trocar at the umbilicus
Excessive force
Blunt trocars
Failure to maintain perpendicular entry with secondary ports
Obesity

reported incidence of vascular injury. Standardisation of databases would help overcome this problem.

Surface anatomy

It is important to identify the location of major vessels prior to insertion of instruments. The umbilicus is not a fixed anatomical landmark. The patient's BMI and the position of the patient affect the location of the umbilicus relative to the bifurcation of the aorta.[13]

The tops of the iliac crests are consistent surface landmarks for the fourth-lumbar vertebrae and, in 80% of cases, the aortic bifurcation will lie within 1.25 cm of L4.[14] The iliac crests are usually still palpable even in obese patients and should be used as the surface markers for the level of the aortic bifurcation rather than the umbilicus.

Position of the patient

There are several factors to consider if trocars or the Veress needle are introduced in the Trendelenburg position as opposed to the supine position (Fig. 1).

Horizontal position

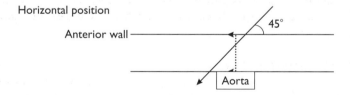

15° Trendelenburg position

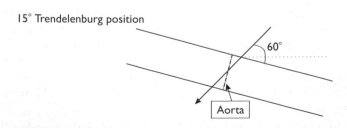

Fig. 1 Effects of Trendelenburg on entry technique.

1. The angle of tilt may be difficult to judge once the surgical drapes are in place.

2. The angle of introduction of the Veress/trocar to the horizontal is smaller than when the patient is horizontal.

3. The aortic bifurcation is more likely to be located caudal to the umbilicus in the Trendelenburg position compared with the supine position.

If these factors are not appreciated, the trocar can inadvertently be introduced at a more perpendicular angle, to the patient's longitudinal axis, resulting in an increased chance of damaging the major vessels.

Adequate pneumoperitoneum

In the past, fixed volumes of gas, such as 2–3 l, were advocated to achieve adequate pneumoperitoneum. However, the size of the abdominal cavity and distensiability of the abdominal wall are variable; 3 l of CO_2 may cause minimal distension in a large patient. The intra-abdominal pressure is now regarded as a more reliable guide to insufflation.

An intra-abdominal pressure of 20 mmHg is associated with a reliable elevation of the anterior abdominal wall. This should reduce the risk of injury to the great vessels. The pressure should be reduced to 12–15 mmHg once the trocars have been inserted.[11,12]

Lifting the abdominal wall

Some surgeons advocate mechanical elevation of the abdominal wall during insertion of the Veress needle. This increases the distance to the great vessels; however, there is evidence it may increase the risk of pre peritoneal insufflation of gas, which may then complicate the entry procedure.[15]

Open laparoscopy

Performing open laparoscopy will reduce the incidence of vascular injury during introduction of the primary trocar; however, it does not eliminate the risk. Cases of trauma to the aorta have been reported.[16] The risk of bowel injury is discussed later.

Vascular injury and secondary trocars

Secondary trocars used in gynaecological surgery are normally sited in the lower half of the abdomen. It is important to identify the inferior and the superficial epigastric vessels. The inferior epigastric artery arises from the external iliac artery and anastomoses with the superior epigastric artery. It lies between the rectus sheath muscle and the peritoneum. The inferior epigastric artery may be identified by direct visualisation; a common mistake is to identify the obliterated hypogastric artery as the inferior epigastric artery. The inferior epigastric artery usually lies 1–2 cm lateral to the obliterated hypogastric artery, but the position of these vessels does vary and the obliterated vessels may not be identifiable in patients who have had previous surgery or in the obese.

The superficial epigastric vessels arise from the femoral vessels near the inguinal ring and course, over the rectus muscle, toward the umbilicus. In thin patients, they can be identified by transillumination; however, in obese patients, the vessels may not identified.

It is important to introduce the secondary trocars at 90° to the skin. If this angle is not maintained, the trocar may deviate from the preselected site and could result in vascular trauma. In the event of vascular trauma, the trocar sleeve should be left in place as a marker for the injured vessel.

Techniques to repair an injured anterior wall vessel

1. If the vessel ends are visible through the laparoscope, coagulation with diathermy may be possible.

2. Pass a No. 12 Foley catheter through the port, inflate the balloon, remove the port and use the balloon to create a tamponade, which should be maintained for 4–6 h.[17]

3. A ligating suture placed below the injury (or above if venous) should secure haemostasis. Instruments such as the Endoclose (Tyco Health Care) may aid suture placement.

4. If bleeding is brisk, the skin incision around the trocar can be enlarged and both the ends of the vessel dissected out and ligated. It is imperative that both ends of the vessel are ligated because of the anastomoses with the superior epigastric artery.

MINIMISING BOWEL INJURY DURING LAPAROSCOPIC ENTRY

Bowel injuries, occurring during laparoscopic entry, have been classified into two groups:[12] type I – damage by the Veress or trocar to normally located bowel; and type II – damage by the Veress or trocar to bowel adherent to the abdominal wall.

In the presence of adhesions, bowel injury during laparoscopic entry is more likely to occur. The risk of adhesions to the abdominal wall is detailed below (Table 3). Procedures have been developed to minimise the risk of type II injuries; these include saline mapping, microlaparoscopy in the left upper quadrant, optical trocars, radially expanding trocars and open laparoscopy.

Table 3 The incidence of peri-umbilical adhesions in relation to previous surgery[18]

Previous surgery	Significant peri-umbilical adhesions (%)
No previous surgery	0.4
Laparoscopy	0.8
Pfannenstiel	6.9
Midline laparotomy	31.5

We are unlikely to produce evidence on which technique is superior as a 33% reduction in bowel injury would require 800,000 cases in a randomised controlled trial.

TECHNIQUES DEVELOPED TO MINIMISE INJURY TO BOWEL INJURY

Saline tests

Once the Veress needle is inserted, 2–3 ml of saline is injected down the Veress needle. It should flow in freely and nothing should be withdrawn if the needle is intraperitoneal. The 'hanging drop test' can also be used to establish if the needle is intraperitoneal; a small drop of saline is placed on the barrel end of the Veress needle, with the tap closed. The anterior abdominal wall is then elevated and the tap of the Veress opened; the negative pressure of the intra-abdominal cavity should cause the drop of saline to flow into the cavity.

Saline mapping

Once pneumoperitoneum is established, saline mapping should be performed prior to inserting the primary trocar; 10 ml of saline injected in an arc below the umbilicus should flow in freely, and only gas should be withdrawn. This is simple and quick to perform and can, therefore, be used in all cases. If brown or turbid fluid is aspirated, the presence of bowel under the umbilicus should be suspected, in which case a 2 mm or 5 mm laparoscope should be inserted at Palmer's point or the procedure abandoned. Palmer's point is found in the left upper quadrant of the abdomen, in the midclavicular line, 3 cm below the costal margin. Prior to using Palmer's point, the possibility of splenomegally should be considered.

Microlaparoscopy

Factors that increase the risk of adhesions to the abdominal wall include a past history of abdominal surgery, peritonitis, endometriosis, or pelvic inflammatory disease.

Audebert[18] inserted a microlaparoscope (a laparoscope less than 2 mm in diameter) at Palmer's point in 814 women undergoing laparoscopy, to study the incidence of peri-umbilical adhesions in relation to previous surgery. The results are summarised in Table 3. In view of these findings, Audebert recommended microlaparoscopy at Palmer's point in women with a previous laparotomy.

Open laparoscopy

Since Hasson[19] developed the technique of open laparoscopy in 1971, it has been accepted more readily by general surgeons than by gynaecologists. A slightly larger incision is required at the umbilicus with sharp dissection down to the peritoneum to allow direct entry into the peritoneal cavity. The approach does appear to reduce type 1 bowel and vascular injuries. However, evidence is conflicting on reduction of type II injuries (where there are adhesions), which vary between 0.2 and 12/1000 (Table 4).

Table 4 Incidence of visceral and vascular trauma following open laparoscopy

Study	Year	Number of cases	Visceral trauma	Vascular trauma
Hasson et al.[20]	2000	5284	0.2/1000	0
Penfield[21]	1985	10,840	0.6/1000	Not stated
Levy et al.[22]	1984	8000	12/10000	0

The sizes of the published series of open laparoscopy are much smaller than the closed laparoscopic techniques. In view of the low incidence of complications, the generalisabilty of the results of the 'open' studies is less certain. The open technique can also be associated with a significant degree of gas leakage during the procedure. This can make visualisation of the operating field more difficult and may, in turn, lead to increased operative complications.

Closed laparoscopy may result in less severe trauma to bowel than open laparoscopy. Bateman et al.[23] reported 6 cases of peri-umbilical adhesions, 3 were diagnosed during the saline aspiration test during closed laparoscopy. In these cases, a laparotomy was avoided. Of the three cases identified during open laparoscopy, in one the bowel was opened and a laparotomy was required.

Direct insertion of the trocar

In 1978, Dingfelder[24] proposed direct insertion of the trocar into the peritoneal cavity. This is a rapid technique, but may be associated with a higher risk of type II bowel injury. However, this risk is not apparent when used in a population with a low risk of adhesions.[11]

Optical trocars

Trocars have been manufactured which allow visualisation of the abdominal wall layers during introduction of the trocar into the peritoneal cavity. There is no evidence that they reduce type II injuries to bowel.

Others

In the past, some surgeons advocated swinging the Veress needle in an arc under the umbilicus to establish if it is free. This practice is not recommended as it may convert a small needle injury to the bowel into a significant tear.

MANAGEMENT OF BOWEL INJURIES

If the Veress needle has been inserted into bowel with no tearing, then conservative management, antibiotics and observation appear to be appropriate.[23] If the trocar has penetrated bowel, it is best left in place to mark the injury. Some injuries can be repaired laparoscopically, whilst others will require a laparotomy.

Bishoff et al.[25] conducted a review of bowel complications; over 69% of bowel injuries are not recognised at the time of surgery. They usually become apparent 12–36 h after surgery, by which time patients may have been discharged. Delayed presentation up to 29 days post-surgery has been reported. Trauma to small bowel tends to present earlier than trauma to large bowel.[25] Thermal injuries to the bowel tend to present later than non-thermal injuries. This is probably due to delayed tissue necrosis around the injury.[26]

Histologically, it is possible to distinguish thermal and sharp 'trocar' injuries.

Presentation of bowel trauma can be subtle and different from those associated with classic faecal peritonitis. Persistent pain around a single trocar site, diarrhoea and abdominal distension have all been reported. Diffuse abdominal pain, ileus, nausea and vomiting are rare symptoms. The white cell count may not be elevated, there may even be leukopaenia.[25]

Postoperative pyrexia is unusual following laparoscopic surgery and should be regarded with great suspicion. All patients should be advised to return to the hospital if they develop worsening pain. Gynaecologists should have a high index of suspicion for bowel injuries following laparoscopic surgery.

EFFECT OF BMI ON LAPAROSCOPIC ENTRY

Low BMI
In patients with a low BMI, the great vessels can lie as little as 2.5 cm below the umbilicus.[27] In this group, the abdominal wall should be elevated and the Veress should be held on the shaft not the barrel[11] thereby increasing the distance from the umbilicus to the aorta and reducing the length of needle to be inserted.

High BMI
In obese patients, there is an increased risk of preperitoneal insertion of the Veress needle due to the increased thickness of their abdominal wall. Hurd *et al.*[28] assessed the depth of insertion of the Veress required to reach the peritoneal cavity in patients with a BMI > 30, in relation to the method of insertion. The results are shown in Table 5.

Table 5 The depth of insertion of the Veress required to reach the peritoneal cavity in patients with a BMI > 30[28]

Incision	Peri-umbilical at 45° to the skin	Umbilical base at 45°	Umbilical base at 90°
Distance from incision to peritoneal cavity	16 cm	11 cm	< 6 cm

The average distance from the base of the umbilicus to the aorta in obese women was 13 cm. In the obese patient, it may be appropriate to introduce the Veress needle through the base of the umbilicus at 90° to the skin. This increases the chance of achieving pneumoperitoneum without compromising the risk of vascular injury.

CONCLUSIONS

Entry techniques should possibly be tailored to the individual patient because there is no conclusive evidence as to the safest entry technique in all circumstances. In 1999, an international group of gynaecologists and surgeons with an interest in laparoscopic surgery compiled a consensus document on laparoscopic entry techniques.[12] The proposals are summarised in Box 2.

REDUCING EXIT COMPLICATIONS OF LAPAROSCOPY

VASCULAR COMPLICATIONS

During laparoscopy, the pressure maintained within the abdominal cavity may produce a tamponade effect on venous bleeding. It is, therefore, advisable to reduce the pressure and observe the operating field at the end of the procedure

Box 2 Entry technique for closed laparoscopy proposed in the consensus document 1999

Identify risks of bowel adhesion

If at high risk of bowel adhesion, exclude splenomegaly and introduce a microlaparoscope at Palmer's point

Ensure the bladder is empty

Check the abdomen for masses and the position of the aorta

Many feel the patient should be horizontal during all entry procedures

Primary incision should be made, through the skin only, at the base of the umbilicus

Check the Veress is sharp, has a good spring action and allows gas to flow

The umbilicus should be elevated during insertion of the Veress

Insertion of the Veress should stop as soon as the peritoneal cavity is entered

Tests (saline aspiration, gas flow-pressure readings) should be performed to establish the Veress is in the peritoneal cavity

The Veress needle should **NOT** be swung under the peritoneum

CO_2 should be insufflated to 25 mmHg until all trocars are inserted

The primary trocar should be introduced through the base of the umbilicus

Once the laparoscope is inserted, a 360° survey should be performed to exclude bowel or vascular trauma

prior to removing the laparoscope.[29] The trocar sheaths can also have a tamponade effect on damaged vessels at the site of port incisions. Each incision should be visualised after the sheath has been removed.

BOWEL TRAUMA

Rapid release of the pneumoperitoneum in conjunction with removal of a port may result in a loop of bowel being sucked into the incision. Removal of all ports should be visualised. During removal of the umbilical port, the laparoscope should protrude from the port during its removal.[30]

INCISIONAL HERNIA

The incidence of port-site herniation varies up to 0.2%. In 86% of cases, the port site was greater than or equal to 10 mm. The fascial layer should be closed in all incisions greater than 10 mm to minimise the risk of hernia.[31]

MINIMISING THE COMPLICATIONS OF ELECTROSURGERY

The incidence of electrosurgical complications during laparoscopic surgery is difficult to ascertain. The most commonly injured structure is bowel. Other injuries reported include ureteral strictures, hydroureter, and fistula formation.

The risk of electrosurgery can be minimised through understanding the principles of the technology. Electrosurgery is the passage of high-frequency electrical current through tissue, that generates heat, to cut or coagulate tissue. Normal mains electrical current causes cell damage by irreversible depolarisation of the cell membrane, but the diathermy generator avoids this because the current frequency is very high. This is in contrast to electrocautery in which the surgical instrument is heated by passage of current through it; the heat of the instrument is then transferred to the tissue.

Factors that influence the diathermy effect are current density, the resistance of the tissue, the waveform and the duration of activation.

At high current density, heat is produced. The size of the electrode influences current density. At the tip of an active electrode, the current density is high hence heat is generated. Increasing the area of electrode in contact with the tissue will reduce the current density and the heating effect.

Cutting is achieved by using a low voltage but a high frequency current that is constantly flowing. The current is concentrated in a very small area and the high-energy level causes cells to explode releasing steam. If coagulation is required, then an intermittent high-voltage current is used, with current only flowing for about 6% of the time. Thus, a cutting current is inherently safer because of the lower voltage reducing the risk of inadvertent current discharge through insulation failure. The mechanisms of electrosurgical injury are summarised in Box 3.

Box 3 Mechanisms of electrosurgical injury

Accidental application
Misidentification of anatomy
Distant site burns
Insulation failure
Direct coupling
Capacitance coupling

Accidental application
Situations that increase the risk of accidental application include the operating surgeon not activating the power supply to the instrument and operating on a mobile structure which is not adequately stabilised, for example an ovarian cyst. Spirit-based skin preparation products used in close proximity to diathermy can result in burns.

Misidentification of anatomy
This is self-evident, but one should also consider the relative proximity of other structures. The effects of diathermy can spread to underlying structures, for example the ureter underlying endometriosis on the pelvic side-wall. The field of view in endoscopic surgery is smaller than open surgery, which increases the risk of out-of-view injury.

Distant-site burns
The safety of electrosurgical equipment is continually improving. The introduction of solid-state generators in 1968 meant that current would only flow if it was returning to the generator. This avoided distant-site burns cause

by concentration of current at alternative sites such as a drip stand touching the patient. However, return electrode burns could still occur if the return pad was not fully attached. Systems of contact quality monitoring are available to prevent return electrode burns.

If an electrosurgical instrument is not producing the desired effect, one should always check the circuit and not automatically increase the power.

The use of bipolar diathermy removes the need for a distant electrode and the active and return electrodes are only millimetres apart. It is an inherently safer form of diathermy.

Direct coupling

This is the flow of current from one instrument to another. It may be secondary to insulation failure or inadvertent discharge to a non-insulated instrument. When using diathermy, all instruments should be insulated.

Insulation failure

This is due to damaged equipment. The risk of insulation failure is increased if high-voltage coagulation settings are used. The use of disposable equipment is claimed to reduce the incidence of insulation failure, but some disposable instruments may be less robust than re-usable instruments and they can be damaged even during a single case, particularly if prolonged. Insulation damage caused by the repeated trauma of passing the instrument through a port is a particular hazard.

Capacitance coupling

A capacitor is formed by two conductors separated by an insulator; for example, an insulated laparoscopic instrument passing through a metal port. The current stored in the capacitor can discharge into the patient causing burns. The higher the current passing through the active instrument, the greater will be the capacitance current. Plastic ports do not eliminate the risk of capacitance coupling because the patient's bowel can act as the second conductor. Active electrode monitoring systems can avoid capacitance coupling.

Electrosurgical injuries to bowel

The majority of electrosurgical injuries to the bowel are unrecognised at the time of surgery.[32] There can be considerable delay before the symptoms of bowel perforation become apparent following electrosurgical injury.[25]

Harmonic scalpel

Ultrasound is the basis for the energy used in the harmonic scalpel. The blade of the scalpel vibrates at 55.5 kHz causing denaturation of proteins and providing coagulation at 50–100°C, a lower temperature than diathermy. This is associated with less charring and smoke. It does not have the risk of aberrant electrical current discharge. No peer-reviewed clinical trials have compared the harmonic scalpel and electrosurgery.

MINIMISING LEGAL REPERCUSSIONS OF MEDICAL COMPLICATIONS

The primary aim of this article is the reduction of complications of minimal access surgery to the patient. However, all surgical procedures should be performed in expectation of benefit, but with the realisation of risk of harm. No matter how meticulous the surgeon, complications will occur. Pre-operatively, patients should understand the risks of a procedure and the possible complications. Possible risks should be discussed in absolute numerical terms rather than qualitative terms such as small, slight, or rare. 'Material risk' is increasingly being used to assess if consent was adequate.

A risk is material if: 'in the circumstances of the case, a reasonable person in the patient's position, if warned of the risk, would be likely to attach significance to it or if the medical practitioner is, or should reasonably be aware that the particular patient if warned of the risk, would be likely to attach significance to it'.[32]

In practice, this implies that even rare complications that are serious or that carry significance to an individual's social life or employment should be addressed.

Key points for clinical practice

- Although the incidence of major complications during laparoscopy is low, laparoscopy is a widely used procedure and 75 women in the UK each year will sustain a major complication.

- There is no evidence that one entry technique is safer or more successful than another in all patients. However, there is a published consensus of professional opinion about safe practice.

- In closed laparoscopy, a saline test may help to prevent trocar injuries to the bowel.

- Secondary ports should be introduced under direct vision.

- Surgeons should understand the principles of electrosurgery.

- Material risk should be considered when obtaining consent from patients.

References

1. Chapron C, Fauconnier A, Goffinet F, Breart G, Dubuisson J. Laparoscopic surgery is not inherently dangerous for patients presenting with benign gynaecological pathology. *Hum Reprod* 2002; **17**: 1334–1342.
2. Kreb H. Intestinal injury in gynecological surgery: a ten year experience. *Am J Obstet Gynecol* 1986; **155**: 509–514.
3. Wittgen C, Andrus C, Fitzgerald S. Analysis of haemodynanic and ventilatory effects of laparoscopic cholecystectomy. *Arch Surg* 1991; **126**: 997–1000.
4. Joris J. Anaesthetic management of laparoscopy. In: Miller RD (ed) *Anaesthesia*. Edinburgh: Churchill Livingstone, 1994: 2011–2029.
5. Safran D, Sgambati S, Orlando R. Laparoscopy in high risk cardiac patients. *Surg Gynecol Obstet* 1993; **176**: 548–554.
6. Mintz M. Risks and prophylaxis in laparoscopy: survey of 100,000 cases. *J Reprod Med* 1977; **18**: 269–272.
7. Loffer F, Pent D. Indications, contra-indications and complications of laparoscopy. *Obstet Gynecol Surv* 1975; **30**: 407–423.

8. Bergqvist D, Bergqvist A. Vascular injuries during gynaecological surgery. *Acta Obstet Gynaecol* 1987; **66**: 19–23.

9. Chapron C, Querleu D, Bruhat M *et al*. Surgical complications of diagnostic and operative gynaecological laparoscopy: a series of 29 966 cases. *Hum Reprod* 1998; **13**: 867–872.

10. Harkki-Siren P, Sjoberg J, Kurki T. Major complications of laparoscopy: a follow-up Finnish study. *Obstet Gynecol* 1999; **94**: 94–98.

11. Garry R. Towards evidence-based laparoscopic entry techniques: clinical problems and dilemmas. *Gynaecol Endosc* 1999; **8**: 315–326.

12. Anon. A consensus document concerning laparoscopic entry techniques: Middlesborough, March 19–20. *Gynaecol Endosc* 1999; **8**: 403–406.

13. Hurd W, Bude R, Delancey J, Pearl M. The relationship of the umbilicus to the aortic bifurcation: implications for laparoscopic technique. *Obstet Gynecol* 1992; **81**: 48–51.

14. Gray H. *Anatomy of the Human Body*, 28th edn. Philadelphia, PA: Lea Febiger; 1966.

15. Briel J, Plaiser P, Meijer W, Lange J. Is it necessary to lift the abdominal wall when preparing a pneumoperitoneum? A randomized study. *Surg Endosc* 2000; **14**: 862–864.

16. Hanney R, Carmalt H, Merrett N, Tait N. Use of the Hasson cannula producing major vascular injury at laparoscopy. *Surg Endosc* 1999; **13**: 1238–1240.

17. Corfman R, Diamond M, DeCherney A. *Complications of Laparoscopy and Hysteroscopy*. Oxford: Blackwell, 1993.

18. Audebert AJGV. Role of microlaparoscopy in the diagnosis of peritoneal and visceral adhesions and the prevention of bowel injury associated with blind trocar insertion. *Fertil Steril* 2000; **73**: 631–635.

19. Hasson H. A modified instrument and method for laparoscopy. *Am J Obstet Gynecol* 1971; **110**: 886–887.

20. Hasson HM, Rotman C, Rana N, Kumari NA. Open laparoscopy: 29-year experience. *Obstet Gynecol* 2000; **96**: 763–766.

21. Penfield A. How to prevent complications of open laparoscopy. *J Reprod Med* 1985; **30**: 660–663.

22. Levy B, Hulka J, Peterson H, Phillips J. Operative laparoscopy: American Association of Gynecologic Laparoscopist 1993 Membership Survey. *J Am Assoc Gynecol Laparosc* 1994; **1**: 301–305.

23. Bateman B, Kolp L, Hoeger K. Complications of laparoscopy – operative or diagnostic. *Fertil Steril* 1996; **66**: 30–35.

24. Dingfelder J. Direct trocar insertion without prior pneumoperitoneum. *J Reprod Med* 1978; **21**: 45–47.

25. Bishoff J, Allaf M, Kirkels W, Moore R, Kavoussi L, Schroder F. Laparoscopic bowel injury: incidence and clinical presentation. *J Urol* 1999; **161**: 887–890.

26. Levy B, Soderstrom R, Dail D. Bowel injuries during laparoscopy: gross anatomy and histology. *J Reprod Med* 1985; **30**: 168–172.

27. Hulka J. Major vessel injury during laparoscopy. *Am J Obstet Gynecol* 1980; **138**: 590.

28. Hurd W, Bude R, Delancey J, Gauvin J, Aisen A. Abdominal wall characteristics by MRI and CT imaging: the effect of obesity on laparoscopic approaches. *J Reprod Med* 1991; **36**: 473–476.

29. Broome J, Lamaro V, Vancaillie T. Changes in hemostatic mechanisms associated with operative laparoscopy. *J Am Assoc Gynecol Laparosc* 2000; **7**: 149–153.

30. Clarke T, Byrne D. The port-decompression effect. A causative factor in the aetiology of post-laparoscopic port-site herniation? *Gynaecol Endosc* 2000; **9**: 181–184.

31. Nezhat C, Nezhat F, Seidman D, Nezhat C. Incisional hernias after laparoscopy. *J Laparoendosc Adv Surg Tech* 1997; **7**: 111–115.

32. Tucker R, Voyles C. Laparoscopic electrosurgical complications and their prevention. *AORN J* 1995; **62**: 49–78.

33. Rogers v Whitaker. In: CRL; 1992, 479.

Patrick Hogston

13

Advances in the surgical management of vaginal prolapse

A renewed interest in surgery for vaginal prolapse has developed in recent years with the use of the term 'pelvic reconstructive surgery' helping to place the emphasis on the aim of prolapse surgery – namely the restoration of structure and function. Much of the scientific literature on pelvic reconstructive surgery consists of uncontrolled observational studies of one technique for a limited period of time. Controlled or randomised studies are rare but where available will be the basis of this review, along with recent studies reporting long-term outcomes.

ANATOMY

The basis of all surgery is a thorough knowledge of anatomy. There has been considerable debate on the relative importance of fascia and muscles. Many of the operations performed to improve prolapse are largely based on the theory that support structures were stretched and thus needed to be shortened and plicated and that the vagina was stretched rather than being displaced. Therefore, excision of this 'excess' vaginal skin is common practice. Other operations compensate for abnormal anatomy such as the placement of levator stitches in the posterior repair. Our understanding of anatomy has increased in recent years partly from rediscovering earlier work. In 1972, Baden and Walker[1] argued that prolapse was not due to stretching, but rather breaks in fascia which could and should be identified and repaired individually. Fresh cadaver dissection and magnetic resonance imaging (MRI) have helped to clarify the fascial supports of the vagina and their attachments to the pelvic side wall.[2] Biochemical studies have shown that the collagen in postmenopausal women with prolapse shows a change in metabolism resulting in a significant alteration in the balance between type I (strongest) and type III (more elastic).[3]

Patrick Hogston BSc (Hons) FRCS FRCOG, Consultant Gynaecologist, St Mary's Hospital, Milton Road, Portsmouth PO3 6AD, UK

Details of muscular and fascial supports have been demonstrated on MRI of healthy nulliparous women. As support of the vagina is both muscular and fascial, defects in one or both could be possible. In the case of rectocoele, the fascia may be defective because of lack of support by the levator ani. It has been suggested that the success rate for rectocoele repair may depend more on the strength of the levator ani than on the technique of repair.

However, what we need to know is whether operations work and whether they cause any specific problems rather than necessarily changing the technique of the operation just because we no longer believe them to be anatomically correct.

Petros[4] has recently studied the anatomy in 50 patients with prolapse using radio-opaque dye in the bladder, vagina and rectum and in an additional 12 patients by injecting it into the levator plate. He then performed lateral standing X-rays in the resting and straining position. Perineal ultrasound was also performed. Seven nullipara acted as controls. The posterior vaginal wall was stretched backwards and rotated downward against the perineal body with straining. Petros postulates that the fascial structures in level 2 transmit the contractile forces of the levator plate to stretch and angulate the vagina backwards. Lax connective tissue may thus prevent this. The perineal body needs to be strong to allow angulation around it. As a result of these studies, Petros proposed a new technique for vault prolapse to re-inforce all three levels of support which will be discussed later.

SURGICAL PRINCIPLES AND MATERIALS

Collagen is central to wound healing and the weaker, more elastic type III is laid down first. With maturation, type I replaces type III but the new tissue is never as strong as the original. Fascia will only have regained 15% of its original strength by 14 days and takes 3 months to regain 70%.[3] However, the commonest sutures used for vaginal repair are rapidly absorbable materials such as polyglycollic acid and polyglactin. Hence, first principles should tell surgeons to use a longer-acting material even though this has not formally been tested by a randomised controlled trial. Gynaecologists have perhaps been slow in utilising the newer synthetic sutures now available and have relied on the inflammatory response of older materials. Materials that last 3 weeks will not help fascia to regain its strength. How much this might influence the recurrence of vaginal prolapse is not proven. If the analogy with herniae is used and prolapse is due to breaks in fascial supports, then it is clear from results with hernia repair that only delayed absorbable or permanent sutures should be used. However, permanent sutures in the vagina cause problems with infection, granulations, bleeding and even fistula formation and may require removal. Delayed absorbable sutures may be a better option, but this is an area that clearly requires further study. For recurrent prolapse surgery including sacrospinous fixation, absorbable, delayed and non-absorbable sutures have been used. Observational data suggest that permanent sutures such as braided polyester, polypropylene or polytetrafluoroethylene (PTFE) give improved results.[5] However, data in hernia repair suggest an increased risk of infection with PTFE compared with monofilament sutures. More data on suture material in pelvic reconstructive surgery are required.

TRIALS IN SURGERY

Surgery for prolapse is reconstructive and, as with all other surgical reconstruction, has a recognised and indeed expected failure rate even when strong artificial material is used, such as in orthopaedic surgery. It is not really surprising that pelvic reconstructive surgery for prolapse will also have a failure rate. Surgery cannot correct the muscle and nerve damage that is part of the aetiology and cure rates are likely to be worse the more severe the prolapse being treated.

Surgical research has largely consisted of retrospective case series or observational data of a new technique with occasional reference to historical controls to show that the new technique is nearly always better.

McCullogh et al.[6] have addressed the argument that only randomised controlled trials are valid methods of comparing treatments. Randomised controlled trials present special difficulties in surgery, but have been performed. Randomisation between surgeons may be one option but, although this was the methodology used in the trial showing the superiority of colposuspension over anterior repair in the treatment of stress incontinence, it is a method that is rarely used. Funding of surgical trials is a difficulty, but trials of new graft materials in prolapse surgery are perfectly feasible and could be part funded by the manufacturing companies.

FASCIAL DEFECT REPAIR

Baden and Walker[1] identified a 30% failure rate of surgery and after cadaver dissections proposed that **breaks** in the fascia, rather than stretching, could account for all defects. They proposed that these breaks should be identified and repaired individually when treating prolapse surgically. This particularly applied to anterior wall defects where fascia could be torn either laterally from the arcus tendineus, centrally or both. Similarly, with posterior wall defects, the fascia is often detached from the perineal body although central and lateral tears also occur. However, the existence of vaginal fascia has been the subject of considerable controversy with some even denying its existence. Identification at surgery, particularly with large long standing defects is difficult.

In cases of uterine prolapse, the uterosacral ligaments may be detached from the cervix or torn near their sacral attachment. If one accepts the above argument and the technique can be shown to give better results than previous methods, then the surgical challenge is finding these defects during surgery. This will radically change the way prolapse surgery is performed. Lateral defects of the anterior wall have been identified on MRI, but this is less easy with other defects. Richardson was the first to report abdominal paravaginal repair for cystocoele and stress incontinence, but this was an uncontrolled, observational subjective study without urodynamics and a later randomised comparison with longer follow-up has cast considerable doubt on its efficacy as a treatment for urinary stress incontinence.[7] This shows that changes in surgical practice cannot be made until proper comparative studies are performed and that new techniques are clearly not always better. Many surgeons have thus waited to see better evidence before making a complete change in their surgical technique.

ANTERIOR VAGINAL WALL PROLAPSE

The literature on methods of anterior vaginal wall repair have been reviewed by Weber and Walters.[8] They concluded that dissection during anterior colporrhaphy splits the vaginal muscularis and adventitia in the midline which may pull the lateral attachments further from the pelvic side-wall. Reported failure rates for anterior repair range from 0–20% and for paravaginal repair from 3–14%. Controlled comparative studies are required to address whether paravaginal repair is required for the treatment of cystocoele in the presence of lateral defects (see below).

POSTERIOR VAGINAL WALL PROLAPSE

Traditional rectocoele repair is associated with a high incidence of dyspareunia probably as a result of a faulty anatomical basis. Most standard texts discuss plication of the levator muscles. However, this is likely to be the cause of dyspareunia and is not necessary. Kahn and Stanton[9] showed that this technique only reduced prolapse symptoms by 50% and increased sexual dysfunction from 18% to 27%. Fascial defect repairs have only been reported in observational uncontrolled studies. Outcomes on over 300 patients followed for a minimum of 6 months have been reported in a variety of retrospective studies from the US and Scandinavia. For example, Porter et al.[10] showed a significant improvement in POP-Q scores as well as symptoms of protrusion, difficult defaecation and constipation ($P < 0.05$) and aspects of daily living ($P < 0.05$). The effect on sexual function was more varied with improvements in the majority (70–90%), but worsened or occurred de novo dyspareunia in up to 19%. Recurrence rates are not clear. Evidence that a change in technique for rectocoele repair improves outcomes is, therefore, more apparent.

GRAFT MATERIALS

Supporting structures in women with prolapse are weak and, therefore, the use of a graft material to give added support is attractive. Evidence from meta-analysis for open groin hernia repairs concluded that mesh repair is associated with fewer recurrences than non-mesh repair (1.4% versus 4.4%; $P < 0.001$).[3] Unfortunately, prolapse repair surgery has a much higher recurrence rate and mesh repair has potentially more complications than when used for herniae. Graft material can be naturally occurring or synthetic (Tables 1 and 2) and, to date, have been primarily used for the treatment of stress incontinence (e.g. Aldridge fascial sling) and in abdominal sacrocolpopexy using synthetic mesh. Their use in the vagina has been limited due to adverse effects. These include infection, rejection, and fibrosis leading to subsequent dyspareunia and thus failing to maintain vaginal function. However, much of the infection may be related to multifilament suture used for fixation rather than the mesh itself. The ideal material would be consistent in strength and quality, available in adequate sizes, easy to handle, and hold sutures. It would be resistant to host absorption, have a low risk of erosion and inflammation, and be available at reasonable cost. Several materials are now available, although none have been shown to meet all of these requirements.

Table 1 Common synthetic biomaterials

Chemical component	Trade names	Type
Polypropylene	Marlex (Bard), Prolene (Ethicon)	Monofilament
Polytetrafluoroethylene (PTFE)	Gore-Tex (Gore), Teflon (Bard)	Multifilament
Polyethylene tetraphthalate	Mersilene (Ethicon)	Multifilament
Polyglycolic acid	Dexon (Davis & Geck)	Multifilament
Polyglactin 910	Vicryl (Ethicon)	Multifilament

Table 2 Available graft materials

Component	Tradename	Source
Patient's fascia	N/A	Patients Rectus, Fascia Lata
Cadaveric fascia	Suspend (Mentor)	Human Cadaveric Fascia Lata
Dermis	Alloderm (Lifecell), Axis (Mentor)	Human
Acellular collagen matrix	Pelvicol (Bard), FortaPerm (Organogenesis)	Porcine
Small intestine submucosa	Surgisis (Cook)	Porcine

AUTOLOGOUS GRAFTS

Autologous fascia

Autologous fascia can be harvested from the rectus fascia or fascia lata. However, it requires an extra wound with an additional site for pain, sepsis, discomfort, operating time, and cosmesis. In addition, there will be a question as to the strength of the patient's own tissue given that prolapse and incontinence may be due to collagen defects. However, there will not be a problem with rejection. Loss of strength with time and shrinkage does occur and they have not been widely used in vaginal reconstructive surgery.

Cadaveric fascia

Freeze dried and solvent dehydrated cadaveric fascia is commercially available (Suspend™) and used in the US, again mostly as sub-urethral slings for women with stress incontinence. Gamma irradiation inactivates transmissible pathogens but this fascia is not used in the UK.

SYNTHETIC GRAFTS

Synthetic materials were also initially used for suburethral slings, but are now widely used for abdominal sacrocolpopexy. There are many different types of mesh which are classified by their pore size. Type 1 (macroporous) meshes contain large pores (> 75 μm) and allow fibroblasts, blood vessels and collagen into the pores. Polyethylene (Mersilene™) and polypropylene (Marlex™, Prolene™) are type 1 meshes that are interwoven and act as a trellis into which patient's own fibro-elastic tissue can grow and galvanise the repair. Marlex™ is a more rigid material and erosion is a potential problem. The fibrosis leads to major concerns for dyspareunia in sexually active women particularly if the mesh is placed via the vagina. A silicone covered polypropylene mesh is also available (Biomesh™), but there is no evidence that this confers a clinical benefit. Because it is macroporous, monofilament and more flexible, Prolene™ is the most popular and probably has a lower erosion rate although this is difficult to prove.

In 2001, Cervigni and Natale[3] reviewed reports on over 700 patients undergoing abdominal sacrocolpopexy with a variety of synthetic materials. The success rate varied between 68–100% with a mesh erosion rate of 0–10% at any time up to 6 years. This is much less than when the materials were used for sub-urethral slings. The explanation for this is probably the higher tension and compromise in perfusion in sub-urethral slings which worsens with time due to shrinkage of the mesh. Late failures with sacrocolpopexy occur for the same reason. Many patients do not require treatment for erosion although attempts can be made to bury the material again. Mesh removal is rarely indicated and can be difficult.

USE OF SYNTHETIC GRAFTS IN TRANSVAGINAL REPAIR SURGERY FOR ANTERIOR VAGINAL PROLAPSE

As discussed previously, vaginal prolapse should be considered as one or more specific defects in the same way as abdominal wall hernias. Surgical treatment of hernias has moved from permanent sutures to tension-free, non-absorbable mesh as this reduces postoperative pain, recovery time and recurrence rate. Synthetic materials have been reported in the vaginal repair of anterior wall prolapse, particularly recurrent prolapse. Julian[11] compared the efficacy and complications of Marlex™ *versus* standard repair in 24 patients with two or more failed anterior repairs. At 2 years, there were no recurrences with Marlex™ as opposed to 4 recurrences with standard repair (*P* < 0.05). Most other reports are uncontrolled, but show high success rates with mesh repair with up to 3 years follow-up and erosion rates of less than 5% although 13% in the largest series. However, many patients with erosion do not require treatment and hence it seems justifiable to offer mesh to patients with two or more failed operations. Polypropylene mesh is marketed as GyneMesh™ for this purpose although there are no published trials of its use.

The issue of mesh in primary surgery is more controversial, but has been addressed in two randomised studies using polyglactin 910 mesh. Weber *et al.*[12] randomly assigned 114 patients to standard repair, standard repair plus polyglactin 910 (absorbable) mesh or ultralateral repair. Of the study group, 83 patients (76%) attended for follow-up at a mean of 23 months; symptom relief and anatomical cure were statistically the same in the three groups. Some had other surgery performed which was not controlled for. Sand *et al.*[13] randomised 161 patients with cystocoele to the hymenal ring and beyond to treatment by anterior repair with or without the same mesh. Patients with paravaginal defects were excluded. Primary and repeat operations were included and mesh used as a bulking material folded into the colporrhaphy sutures, in the belief that it enhanced and protected the central repair. At 1 year, there were 25% recurrences in the mesh group and 43% in the no-mesh group ($P = 0.02$). However, it was not clear how many underwent further surgery. There is still a significant recurrence rate in surgical treatment of anterior wall prolapse whatever method is used. Whilst patients need to be aware of this, most of them are asymptomatic and do not appear to require further surgery, at least in the short term.

USE OF SYNTHETIC GRAFTS IN TRANSVAGINAL REPAIR SURGERY FOR POSTERIOR VAGINAL PROLAPSE

Sand *et al.*[13] used polyglactin mesh in 119 patients in the above study and found 3 recurrences in the mesh group and 4 without the mesh ($P = 0.66$). The use of Marlex™ mesh in posterior repair has been reported in 4 patients with obstructive defaecation. Three patients reported normal defaecation at 18 months.

A variety of new products are now licensed for use in vaginal repair surgery. At the time of writing, none have any comparative data available.

DERMAL ALLOGRAFTS

Acellular human dermal grafts allow neovascularisation and host tissue incorporation. They are available as Alloderm™ and Axis™, are used in cosmetic surgery, and have been shown to be as strong as fascia lata. However, there are no data for use in vaginal surgery.

ACELLULAR COLLAGEN MATRIX

This material is marketed as Pelvicol™ by Bard and FortaPerm™ by Organogenesis Inc. The manufacturing process converts harvested porcine dermis (from health-maintained, monitored herds which are processed for food) into strong non-allergenic, permanent repair material by removing the fat and cellular material by enzymatic extraction to leave only elastin and collagen. The original 3-dimensional structure of the collagen matrix is maintained and is then cross-linked with hexamethylene di-isocyanate (HMDI) to preserve integrity and resist enzyme attack. It is then vacuum packed and sterilised by gamma irradiation. Porcine and human collagen share the same structure and, because it is acellular, it does not become encapsulated or produce a foreign body reaction and acts as scaffold for host tissue. It has the same strength as polypropylene mesh and can hold sutures. It has been used for pubovaginal slings in the surgical treatment of stress incontinence, anterior and posterior repair, laparoscopic sacrocolpopexy as well as to re-inforce colpocleisis. To date, only uncontrolled observational data are available which will not help to define the true place of this material in the primary repair of vaginal prolapse. Their place in recurrent surgery may be easier and quicker to ascertain although the number of patients having more than two operations in the same compartment is comparatively low.

FREEZE-DRIED PORCINE SMALL INTESTINE SUBMUCOSA (SIS)

This is available in the UK as Surgisis™ from Cook. It is a bioactive and absorbable matrix consisting of collagen, elastin and 'growth factors' obtained from pig small intestine. It allows host tissue in-growth and graft replacement prior to complete degradation. It requires soaking to rehydrate before use and there is no risk of HIV transmission. Dermal allografts have greater thickness at 4 months probably due to persistence of the graft along with in-growth of host tissue in the animal model. The material is marketed, amongst other indications, for 'prolapse tissue support/repair and general tissue repair (pelvic floor/bladder)'. The only data from clinical trials at this time are in abstract form.[14] Twenty patients in two groups underwent anterior repair with or without SIS mesh. At 6 months, the mesh group showed a significantly improved outcome.

COST EFFECTIVENESS IN SURGERY FOR PROLAPSE

Cost-effectiveness analysis measures the net cost of providing a service as well as the effectiveness of the service, summarised by the cost-effectiveness ratio (C/E). In this ratio, all costs are included in the numerator and all health outcomes (benefits less harms) in the denominator. The latter should include the most important clinical outcomes. When any new surgical intervention is introduced, safety, efficacy and effectiveness are evaluated, but in addition cost-effectiveness need to be considered. Artificial collagen materials are all around £350 per sheet and synthetic mesh around £40. The wide-spread introduction of these materials will add significantly to the cost of these operations since at least 38,000 operations for prolapse are carried out in the UK each year. Properly controlled cost-effectiveness studies are required to investigate whether they will give better results and prevent the need for further surgery.

The 42nd RCOG Study Group clearly recommended that new implants should be restricted to patients in research trials, preferably randomised controlled trials with appropriate follow-up. Only when safety and efficacy are reasonably established should marketing be approved.[15]

IS HYSTERECTOMY NECESSARY FOR THE TREATMENT OF UTEROVAGINAL PROLAPSE?

Vaginal hysterectomy with pelvic floor repair is now regarded as the standard operation for uterovaginal prolapse. Women are recommended to complete child-bearing before surgery, although the Manchester repair can be utilised for women who desire further children. However, it is likely that fertility will be reduced by surgery. Other supporting techniques can be used, such as abdominal sacrohysteropexy or vaginal sacrospinous fixation. Successful pregnancy and vaginal delivery have been recorded.

More recently, the need for vaginal hysterectomy has been questioned and sascrospinous fixation or sacrohysteropexy used. A small study comparing sacrospinous fixation with or without hysterectomy was reported by Maher *et al.*[16] After a mean follow-up of 30 months, 56 of an original group of 70 patients showed a 3-fold higher incidence of vault prolapse in the group with uterine conservation, although the power of the study was too small. In addition to the problem of managing women with bleeding following this procedure, it seems that there are no data to support conservation of the uterus at the time of repair for uterine prolapse of grade 2 or more.

NEW APPROACHES TO VAULT PROLAPSE

SUPPORT OF THE VAULT AFTER HYSTERECTOMY

The incidence of vault prolapse after vaginal hysterectomy for prolapse is approximately 12% but only 2% when the indication was other than prolapse.[17] Trials of new methods to improve on this will, therefore, require large numbers of patients. There are several methods described in textbooks as prophylaxis against future vault prolapse, but there have been few comparative studies. Cruikshank and Kovac[18] performed a small, randomised study of McCall's method *versus* the Moscowitz-type closure *versus* simple peritoneal closure only in mostly non-prolapse cases. However, some sacrospinous vaginal fixations and repairs were done for 'secondary indications'. The patients in the McCall's technique had significantly less vault prolapse at 3 years.

In cases of vaginal hysterectomy for uterine prolapse, it may be difficult to identify usable uterosacral-cardinal ligaments and the use of sacrospinous fixation has been proposed. A retrospective case controlled study of 128 patients with advanced uterovaginal prolapse followed up for 4–9 years, compared sacrospinous fixation with McCall's culdeplasty.[19] Vaginal vault prolapse was low in both groups (8% *versus* 5%), but anterior wall prolapse was commoner after sacrospinous fixation (14% *versus* 5%). This procedure also took longer and involved the greater use of blood transfusion (5% *versus* 0). Prophylactic sacrospinous fixation at the time of primary vaginal hysterectomy and repair is, therefore, not recommended.

POST-HYSTERECTOMY VAULT PROLAPSE

Post-hysterectomy vault prolapse is usually associated with enterocoele and other support defects. Surgical treatment is thus complex, carries a greater risk, and is more prone to failure than other types of pelvic reconstructive surgery. It has been suggested that recurrent surgery should be focused on a small number of individuals who have a sufficient case-load to improve their expertise.

UTEROSACRAL VAULT SUSPENSION

McCall's culdeplasty has been shown to be an effective treatment in a series of 693 patients from the Mayo Clinic.[20] Between 1976–1987, 693 patients underwent primary vaginal repair of vault prolapse. Morbidity was low and patients were followed up by postal questionnaire as most lived outside the area. There was an 80% response rate and, after a mean follow-up of 8.8 years, 493 (71.1%) had not required further surgery. Only 36 (5.2%) had undergone another repair, but accurate information was missing on the other 164 (23.7%).

Identification of the uterosacral ligaments can be difficult in cases of previous hysterectomy, not least because of retraction closer to the sacrum. Shull et al.[21] described a technique of high uterosacral ligament suspension to ensure that the remnants of the uterosacral ligaments are identified posterior and medial to the ischial spine as close to the sacrum as possible. It is then necessary to re-attach the ligaments to the pubocervical and rectovaginal fascia to re-establish complete fascial integrity. However, there is concern over the position of the ureter, and ureteric occlusion has been reported in up to 10% of cases. Buller et al.[22] studied the uterosacral ligament in cadavers and concluded that the optimal site for fixation is the intermediate point of the ligament at the level of the ischial spine, 1 cm posterior to its most anterior palpable margin with the ligament on tension. There have been no comparative studies of this operation even though it has become widely used in the US. There is scepticism from many surgeons as to whether this technique is really feasible for total vault eversion.

SACROSPINOUS FIXATION

Other vaginal techniques include fixation of the vagina to the sacrospinous or iliococcygeus ligament. As the latter is easier, Maher et al.[23] performed a matched comparative study of surgeons who performed either SSF or iliococcygeus. This showed a higher patient satisfaction rate with sacrospinous fixation (91% *versus* 78%; $P = 0.1$), although objectively there was no difference. Sacrospinous fixation is the preferred technique in the UK when a vaginal approach is used.

The approach to the sacrospinous ligament has mostly been via a posterior vaginal wall incision and the pararectal space. Goldberg et al.[24] approached it anteriorly via the paravaginal space and seemed to get a deeper vagina and less anterior wall prolapse. They compared 92 patients with a posterior approach and 76 done anteriorly both using two PTFE (Gore-Tex™) sutures. The distance between the introitus and the apex was slightly longer in the anterior group (9.08 cm *versus* 8.33 cm; $P = 0.002$). Furthermore, twice as many patients needed re-operation (15% *versus* 7.6%; $P = 0.01$) in the posterior group. Upper vaginal calibre and sexual function were well preserved in both groups. In a different study, bilateral sacrospinous fixation was carried out in 26 of 40 patients. The authors suggest this required significant judgement to avoid tension and noted three anterior prolapses (1 requiring surgery) in the bilateral group *versus* none in the unilateral group. The study by Benson et al.[25] (see below) also used bilateral sacrospinous fixation, for reasons that are nor clear and achieved poorer results. Bilateral sacrospinous vaginal fixation, therefore, is not recommended on present evidence.

ABDOMINAL *VERSUS* VAGINAL SURGERY

Sacrospinous fixation has been compared with abdominal sacrocolpopexy in a RCT reported by Benson et al.[25] Forty patients underwent abdominal sacrocopopexy and paravaginal repair and 48 bilateral sacrospinous fixation and paravaginal repair with needle suspension of the urethra. The abdominal group appeared to do better than the vaginal group – 58% *versus* 29% optimal with 16% *versus* 33% deemed unsatisfactory. Further surgery was performed in 29% of women in the vaginal group and 16% in the abdominal group. This is at great variance from Hardiman and Drutz's uncontrolled case comparison where recurrent vault prolapse was 1.3% with abdominal and 2.4% with sacrospinous fixation.[26] Furthermore, vaginal surgery by Benson *et al.*[25] consisted of bilateral sacrospinous fixation, a technique which may be inferior to unilateral fixation. Abdominal sacrocolpopexy is more expensive due to a longer operating time and hospital stay, but may be more effective. The incremental cost effectiveness per cure may be as much as US$25,900.[27] Careful selection on clinical grounds is likely to be important in achieving high success rates for both operations.

LAPAROSCOPIC APPROACH

It has been suggested that laparoscopy could be used to identify and tag the uterosacral ligaments. The enterocoele sac is then opened vaginally and excised. The sutures can then be retrieved and used to support the vaginal vault and the pericervical ring reconstructed. The addition of laparoscopy to otherwise vaginal surgery needs to be fully evaluated as there will be added risk.

Sacral colpopexy can also be performed by laparoscopy to good effect. Training is important; many patients are overweight with medical problems and have adhesions from previous surgery. There are no randomised trials of laparoscopic *versus* open sacrocolpopexy.

INTRAVAGINAL SLINGPLASTY (IVS)

Vaginal vault repair is complex and laparoscopic techniques have a long learning curve. A new day-care procedure of infracoccygeal sacropexy has been described by Petros based on his integral theory.[28] An open-knit polypropylene tape is passed using a specially designed IVS tunneler (Tyco Healthcare, USA) through a small perineal incision made lateral and below the anal margin, via the ischiorectal fossa to reach a previously made 5 cm transverse vaginal incision just below the vault. The tape is secured to the vagina and the remnants of the uterosacral ligaments by delayed absorbable sutures. A posterior 'bridge' repair is then performed 'to approximate the laterally displaced rectovaginal fascia towards the midline'. Full thickness longitudinal incisions are made to within 1 cm of the introitus. A delayed absorbable 'tension' suture is placed as laterally as possible into the rectovaginal fascia and run subepithelially as a mattress suture in the rectovaginal space. A second stitch is placed 1 cm below and laterally at the level of the uterosacral with a delayed absorbable suture. The vaginal skin is closed without tension. No pack or catheter is used and patients are generally discharged by 24 h.

Petros[28] reported this technique on 75 patients. Two of 71 had vault prolapse at 1 year and 4 of 40 at 4.5 years. There were 12 of 40 with anterior wall prolapse of whom 8 required surgery. A further series of 93 patients followed a median of 12 months has been reported by Farnsworth.[29] No tapes were rejected, but one intra-operative rectal perforation was repaired transanally without sequelae. One patient has required an abdominal sacrocolpopexy after two failed operations. This procedure is from the Australian Ambulatory Vaginal and Incontinence Surgery (AAVIS.org) group committed to minimally invasive and day-case treatment for prolapse and incontinence. Further results and the experience of other centres are awaited.

POSTOPERATIVE CARE

Research is required into postoperative treatment and convalescence recommendations following prolapse surgery. A national Danish study[30] showed that the sick-leave recommendation varied form 2–12 weeks, median 6 weeks for patients with heavy lifting. The recommended return to intercourse was a median of 4 weeks (range, 0–12 weeks) with a range of 0–24 weeks to restrict strenuous activities. There is little scientific basis to these recommendations which could not be explained by demographic reasons. Variations exist in British practice and there is a need for research in this area.

CYSTOSCOPY AT THE TIME OF VAGINAL SURGERY

Several retrospective observational studies have suggested that routine cystoscopy is useful at detecting cystotomies or intravesical suture placement. In addition, intravenous indigo carmine or methylene blue is injected to assess ureteric patency although such injuries will not always be detected by this method. However the question then arises as to whether this should be performed after every vaginal operation. The management of non-effluence of dye is not always straight forward and several questions remain. How long should one wait for dye to be seen, how reliable is the test, should one try and stent the ureter, which sutures should be removed, and whether this compromises the repair. Routine cystoscopy would not be regarded as standard practice in the UK at this time, but is an area for research.

CONCLUSIONS

Many questions remain to be answered in the field of vaginal surgery. A variety of surgical materials are available which may lead to better outcomes but trials are necessary. For vaginal vault prolapse, the promise of intravaginal slingplasty as a 24-h stay remains to be seen as it is evaluated outside of its centre of origin.

Key points for clinical practice

- Surgery is best delayed until child-bearing is complete.

- Standard treatment for uterovaginal prolapse remains vaginal hysterectomy and repair for women whose family is complete.

- Fascial defect repair of rectocoele appears to give good relief of symptoms and result in less dyspareunia than traditional methods using 'levator sutures'.

- Post-hysterectomy vault prolapse is effectively treated by Mayo culdeplasty, vaginal sacrospinous fixation and abdominal sacrocolpopexy.

- The use of mesh and artificial collagen materials have not been evaluated in controlled clinical trials.

- Surgery for recurrent prolapse should be dealt with by surgeons with a regular practice in prolapse surgery.

References

1. Baden WF, Walker T. *Surgical Repair of Vaginal Defects*. Philadelphia, PA: Lippincott, 1992.
2. Leffler KS, Thompson JR, Cundiff GW *et al*. Attachment of the rectovaginal septum to the pelvic sidewall. *Am J Obstet Gynecol* 2001; **185**: 41–43.
3. Cervigni M, Natale F. The use of synthetics in the treatment of pelvic organ prolapse. *Curr Opin Urol* 2001; **11**: 429–435.
4. Papa Petros PE. Vault prolapse I: Dynamic supports of the vagina. *Int Urogynecol J* 2001; **12**: 292–295.
5. Hogston P. Suture choice in general gynaecological surgery. *Obstetrician Gynaecologist* 2001; **3**: 127–131.
6. McCullogh P, Taylor I, Sasako M, Lovett B, Griffin D. Randomised trials in surgery: problems and possible solutions. *BMJ* 2002; **324**: 1448 1451.
7. Colombo M, Milani R, Vitobello D, Maggioni A. A randomised comparison of Burch colposuspension and abdominal paravaginal defect repair for female stress urinary incontinence. *Am J Obstet Gynecol* 1996; **175**: 78–84.
8. Weber AM, Walters MD. Anterior vaginal prolapse: review of anatomy and techniques of surgical repair. *Obstet Gynecol* 1997; **89**: 311–318.
9. Kahn MA, Stanton SL. Techniques of rectocoele repair and their effects on bowel function. *Int Urogynecol J* 1998; **9**: 37–47.
10. Porter WE, Steele A, Walsh P, Kohli N, Karram MM. The anatomic and functional outcome of defect specific rectocoele repairs. *Am J Obstet Gynecol* 1999; **181**: 1353–1358.
11. Julian TM. The efficacy of Marlex mesh in the repair of severe, recurrent vaginal prolapse of the anterior midvaginal wall. *Am J Obstet Gynecol* 1996; **175**: 1472–1475.
12. Weber AM, Walters MD, Piedmonte MR, Ballard LA. Anterior colporrhaphy: a randomised trial of three surgical techniques. *Am J Obstet Gynecol* 2001; **185**: 1299–1304.
13. Sand PK, Koduri, Lobel RW *et al*. Prospective randomised trial of polyglactin 910 mesh to prevent recurrence of cystocoeles and rectocoeles. *Am J Obstet Gynecol* 2001; **184**: 1357–1362.
14. Digesu GA, Khullar V, Hutchings A, Grey J, Selvaggi L. Acellular collagen matrix: the answer to prevent the recurrence of the anterior vaginal wall prolapse. *Int Urogynecol J* 2001; **12 (Suppl 3)**: Abstract 113.
15. MacLean AB, Cardoza L. (eds) *Incontinence in Women*. London: RCOG Press 2002; 439.
16. Maher CF, Slack MP, Slack MC *et al*. Uterine preservation or hysterectomy at sacrospinous colpopexy for uterovaginal prolapse. *Int Urogynecol J* 2001; **12**: 381–385.
17. Marchionni M, Bracco GL, Checcucci V *et al*. The true incidence of vaginal vault prolapse: thirteen year experience. *J Reprod Med* 1999; **44**: 679–684.
18. Cruikshank SH, Kovac SR. Randomised comparison of three surgical methods used at the time of vaginal hysterectomy to prevent posterior enterocoele. *Am J Obstet Gynecol* 1999; **180**: 859–865.
19. Colombo M, Milani R. Sacrospinous ligament fixation and modified McCall culdeplasty during vaginal hysterectomy for advanced vaginal prolapse. *Am J Obstet Gynecol* 1998; **179**: 13–20.
20. Webb MJ, Aronson MP, Ferguson LK, Lee RA. Post hysterectomy vaginal vault prolapse: primary repair in 693 patients. *Obstet Gynecol* 1998; **92**: 281–285.
21. Shull B, Bachofen G, Kuehl T. A transvaginal approach to repair of apical and other associated sites of pelvic organ prolapse using uterosacral ligaments. Am J Obstet Gynecol 2000; **183**: 1365–1373.
22. Buller JL, Thompson JR, Cundiff GW *et al*. Uterosacral ligament: description of anatomic relationships to optimise surgical safety. *Am J Obstet Gynecol* 2001; **97**: 873–879.
23. Maher CF, Murray CJ, Carey MP, Dwyer PL, Ugoni AM. Iliococcygeus or sacrospinous fixation for vaginal vault prolapse. *Obstet Gynecol* 2001; **98**: 40–44.
24. Goldberg RP, Tomezsko JE, Winkler HA *et al*. Anterior or posterior sacrospinous vaginal vault suspension: long-term anatomic and functional evaluation. *Obstet Gynecol* 2001; **98**: 199–204.
25. Benson JT, Lucente V, McClellan E. Vaginal *versus* abdominal reconstructive surgery for the treatment of pelvic support defects: a prospective randomised study with long term outcome evaluation. *Am J Obstet Gynecol* 1996; **175**: 1418–1422.
26. Hardiman P, Drutz HP. Sacrospinous vault suspension and abdominal colposacropexy:

success rate and complications. *Am J Obstet Gynecol* 1996; **175**: 612–616.

27. Holley RL, Richter HE, Varner RE. Sacrospinous fixation *versus* abdominal sacral colpopexy for posthysterectomy vaginal vault prolapse. *J Pelv Surg* 1999; **5**: 320–324.

28. Papa Petros PE. Vault prolapse II: restoration of dynamic vaginal supports by infracoccygeal sacropexy, an axial day-case vaginal procedure. *Int Urogynecol J* 2001; **12**: 296–303.

29. Farnsworth BN. Posterior intravaginal slingplasty (infracoccygeal sacropexy) for severe posthysterectomy vaginal vault prolapse – a preliminary report on efficacy and safety. *Int Urogynecol J* 2002; **13**: 4–8.

30. Ottesen M, Moller C Kehlet H, Ottesen B. Substantial variability in postoperative treatment and convalescence recommendations following vaginal repair: a nationwide questionnaire study. *Acta Obstet Gynecol Scand* 2001; **80**: 1062–1068.

Rick D. Clayton Desmond P.J. Barton

14

Advances in the treatment of endometrial cancer

Endometrial cancer (EC) is often considered as the gynaecological cancer with a more favourable prognosis because of early presentation with post-menopausal bleeding (PMB). However, stage for stage, EC is at least as lethal as cervical cancer. In the industrialised world, it is a common gynaecological cancer with 3900 cases per year in England and Wales and about 38,000 per year in the US. It is the most common gynaecological cancer in the Western world, whereas cervical cancer is the most common gynaecological cancer in non-industrialised countries. Overall, EC ranks as the eight or ninth most common cause of cancer death in women. In the UK, the management of EC is outlined in the *Guidance on Commissioning Cancer Services* (1999) which recommends that the majority of patients with gynaecological cancer be treated in cancer centres.[1] Central to the management of patients is the multidisciplinary team, which includes the clinical nurse specialist, a dedicated gynaecological pathologist and specialist radiologist.

EPIDEMIOLOGY AND PATHOLOGY

The association of endometrial cancer with a hormonal aetiology, specifically unopposed oestrogen, is well known. However, this does not adequately explain cases occurring in premenopausal patients or in patients many years after the menopause who have not taken HRT. There has been considerable interest in the association between EC and tamoxifen, used not only to treat breast cancer but as a prophylaxis in patients at risk for breast cancer.[2] Most recently, concern has been expressed about prolonged use of combined HRT

Rick D. Clayton MD MRCOG, Fellow in Gynaecological Oncology, The Royal Marsden Hospital, Fulham Road, London SW1 6JJ, UK

Desmond P.J. Barton MD FRCSEd MRCOG FACOG, Consultant Gynaecological Oncologist, The Royal Marsden Hospital, Fulham Road, London SW1 6JJ, UK (for correspondence)

(more than 5 years) and risk of endometrial cancer although this was not found in a more recent study.[3,4] Concern has also been expressed about the oestrogenic content of food.

Much less is known about the genetics of endometrial cancer, but the most common association is with hereditary non-polyposis colorectal cancer (HNPCC), which results from germline mutations in DNA mismatch repair genes. In fact, EC is the second most common cancer associated with HNPCC.

It is important to recognise that EC comprises a range of cancer types from the most common endometrioid endometrial adenocarcinoma (EEA), about which most is known, to the less common clear cell cancer (CCC) and uterine papillary serous cancers (UPSC) which have a worse prognosis. Endometrial cancers also include the endometrial stromal sarcomas (ESS) which arise from the stroma and not the glandular component of the endometrium. These rare endometrial cancers are not associated with the 'risk factors' of the more common EEA. Discussions on endometrial cancer should clearly distinguish these subtypes.

FIGO STAGING

The staging of 'corpus uteri' cancer indicates that assessment of potential sites of metastatic disease is important both for the surgeon and the pathologist. One key component is the presence of lymph node metastasis – including the pelvic and para-aortic nodes and the inguinal nodes. Debate continues about: (i) the diagnostic and therapeutic value of surgical excision of the lymph nodes; (ii) whether there should be a lymph node sampling or a lymph node dissection; and (iii) whether both pelvic and para-aortic lymph nodes should be removed. Indeed, consideration also needs to be given to the underlying endometrial pathology. CCC and UPSC are well known to be associated with disseminated disease at the time of presentation, and nodal metastases are common. These cancers are considered high-grade and only the common EEA is graded along traditional lines. Endometrial stromal sarcomas (both low-grade and high-grade tumours) may also be found to have metastatic disease at surgery. The surgical management of these uncommon endometrial cancers requires a thorough laparotomy and sufficient training and expertise to undertake resection of sites of possible or of known metastatic disease.

MANAGEMENT OF PRIMARY ENDOMETRIAL ENDOMETRIOID ADENOCARCINOMA (EEA)

INITIAL ASSESSMENT

This will include a thorough review of the pathology, usually of an endometrial sample obtained at hysteroscopy or by Pipelle (Laboratoire CCD, Paris, France) sampling. The review should be undertaken by a pathologist with a specialist interest in gynaecological cancer. Key decisions include distinguishing between endometrial dysplasias and well-differentiated EEA, between papillary endometrial adenocarcinoma and UPSC, recognition of CCC, and distinguishing between low- and high-grade ESS. In most cases of

EC, the initial mode of treatment will be surgical. Many patients are elderly, obese and with pre-existing morbidity. A careful pre-operative assessment and evaluation by the anaesthetist is mandatory. Consideration must be given to epidural anaesthesia and to initial postoperative care in a surgical high-dependency unit. Excellent postoperative management care is crucial, especially in the elderly and infirm patient.[5] Surgical management must also give consideration to the vaginal route, and assessment for a vaginal hysterectomy should be made at the time of hysteroscopy. The high-grade and poor prognostic UPSC and CCC should be referred to a cancer centre and operated on by a gynaecological oncologist. The radiological method of choice is MRI and not CT scanning, as it is reported to predict the extent of myometrial and cervical involvement.[6,7] Recently, MRI has been combined with intravenous iron preparations to assess lymph nodes for metastatic disease, but this awaits further evaluation, as does PET scanning.

SURGICAL APPROACH

All patients should have a mechanical bowel preparation before surgery. The usual anti-thrombotic measures should be undertaken, and prophylactic antibiotics given on induction of anaesthesia. The patient should be placed in the Lloyd-Davis position when a laparotomy is being planned, and in a modified or low lithotomy position if vaginal surgery is being undertaken. For laparoscopic-assisted procedures, a similar position can be used and the use of hydraulic leg supports facilitates changing the position of the lower limbs during the vaginal portion of the surgery without re-draping the patient.

Abdominal procedures

In most cases, the procedure involves the taking of peritoneal cytology, a total hysterectomy, bilateral salpingo-oophorectomy and lymph node sampling or dissection of both pelvic and para-aortic regions. This can usually be performed through a high transverse supra-pubic incision or a Maylard incision, the latter giving excellent exposure to the pelvis and lower abdomen. For UPSC (and arguably CCC) the surgery should be considered as that for an ovarian cancer, with a midline incision, thorough lymph node sampling or dissection (or removal of obviously involved lymph nodes) omentectomy possibly and appendicectomy. In obese patients, a panniculectomy can also be performed.

Surgical management of lymph nodes

When a lymph node dissection (or sampling) is planned, it is better to under-take the hysterectomy first in the higher surgical risk patient, and then the lymphadenectomy. The same applies when the uterus is bulky. In rare cases when there is gross uterine disease (*e.g.* tumour invading through the uterine wall), care must be used in handling the uterus, as the uterine body may be avulsed from the cervix.

Unlike cervical cancer, in which therapeutic benefit has been demonstrated for pelvic lymphadenectomy, the therapeutic role of lymphadenectomy in endometrial cancer is not established. Kilgore *et al.*[8] suggested a benefit, with improved survival in patients with node sampling compared with no sampling. However, the decision to remove pelvic nodes was influenced by patient characteristics such as weight and age, which also have prognostic implications. Mohan et al.[9] compared the survival of patients who had undergone a total hysterectomy and bilateral salpingo-oophorectomy (TAHBSO) together with full pelvic lymphadenectomy and had been found to have negative nodes, with published data from other centres which had not employed pelvic lymphadenectomy and found better survival in the group of patients who had undergone lymphadenectomy.

Lymphadenectomy is of clinical importance in directing the use of adjuvant radiotherapy. If the pelvic nodes are found to be uninvolved, then radiotherapy is less likely to be given, whereas, if the lymph node status is not known, the patient is more likely to receive pelvic radiotherapy based on the grade of the tumour and the depth of myometrial invasion. In practice, however, this is not always the case. Despite the presence of negative lymph nodes, 77% of the members of the Society of Gynecologic Oncologists (SGO) would still recommend adjuvant radiotherapy for high-risk (stage 1C and stage 1BG3) tumours.[10]

There have been efforts to identify from pre-operative investigations whether to perform a lymphadenectomy, i.e. to identify those patients who are most likely to have lymph node spread.[11] The inaccuracy of pre-operative pathological grading has led some authors to suggest that the safest policy is to perform lymphadenectomy in all patients.[12] For example, grade 1 histology on an endometrial biopsy is upgraded on review of the hysterectomy specimen in approximately 20% of cases and a FIGO stage 1C lesion will be found in 17% of patients with grade 1 histology, of whom approximately 11% will have pelvic node metastases.[12,13] Alternatively, intra-operative frozen section to assess depth of invasion and tumour grade may be used but it is labour-intensive and is not routine practice in the UK. Some surgeons rely on intra-operative assessment of the opened resected specimen.

As to the extent of the lymphadenectomy, palpation of the lymph nodes is not reliable – in 37% of positive lymph nodes, the size of the metastasis will be less than 2 mm in diameter.[15] Therefore, extensive lymph node sampling or complete pelvic lymphadenectomy has been recommended by some authors.[16] Assuming that the surgeon is trained to perform lymphadenectomy, the limiting factor is the likelihood of complications associated with the procedure and whether these complications are likely to be greater the more extensive the lymphadenectomy. Patient factors, such as obesity and performance status, are also important. It has been suggested by some authors that lymphadenectomy or sampling carries a low and acceptable risk of morbidity,[17] and that systematic lymphadenectomy may be safely accomplished in elderly patients.[18]

Furthermore, when radiotherapy is given after pelvic lymphadenectomy, the morbidity is increased. When pelvic nodes are found to be involved, the incidence of para-aortic lymph node involvement is approximately 32% whereas in the absence of pelvic node involvement the incidence of para-aortic involvement is 2.2%.[19] Approximately 30–40% of patients with positive para-aortic nodes will survive long-term with extended field radiotherapy;[19] therefore, it may be important to know the status of these nodes.

The ASTEC (A Study in the Treatment of Endometrial Cancer) trial is currently underway in the UK and may help to resolve some of the controversy surrounding the therapeutic role of lymphadenectomy. Part of the trial consists of a surgical comparison of a policy of conventional surgery (*i.e.* TAH/BSO) with a policy of conventional surgery with a lymphadenectomy (defined as a 'systematic dissection of the iliac and obturator nodes'; para-aortic sampling is 'at the discretion of the surgeon'). Somewhat confusingly, the trial also accepts lymph node sampling in more difficult surgical patients. The trial, therefore, cannot address the role of para-aortic lympth node sampling in EC.

Vaginal procedures

In the elderly infirm patient with the common endometrial adenocarcinoma, a transvaginal hysterectomy can provide rapid palliation of vaginal bleeding with minimal morbidity. In our opinion, in this type of patient there should not be strenuous attempts made to remove the adnexae, which are rarely a site of metastases. Nevertheless, in experienced hands, transvaginal adnexectomy is feasible and safe. This route of surgery should also be considered in the morbidly obese patient. A combined vaginal approach with a retroperitoneal nodal dissection has also been described.[20] Today, most patients with EEC undergoing a transvaginal hysterectomy will have a laparoscopically assisted procedure, not only to remove or sample the lymph nodes but to ensure that the adnexae are removed.

Laparoscopic procedures

Arguments continue over the advantages and disadvantages of laparoscopic surgery compared with abdominal surgery. In our opinion, both techniques are acceptable in the management of endometrial adenocarcinoma. Case selection is central to surgical management. Patient factors to consider include medical and surgical history, uterine size, degree of uterovaginal descent, and transvaginal accessibility. Patient age and obesity are less important. Operator factors include experience both of the individual surgeon and the team. If it is considered appropriate to sample or remove the lower para-aortic lymph nodes, then it must be recognised that very few gynaecologists/oncologists are trained in this laparoscopic technique.

Laparoscopically assisted vaginal hysterectomy together with laparoscopic pelvic/para-aortic node sampling can achieve comparable results in terms of adequacy of surgery in most patients.[21] Case series have demonstrated reduced in-patient time compared with open procedures, and acceptable morbidity, although laparoscopic procedures in obese women can be difficult. The Gynecologic Oncology Group is currently conducting a prospective randomised trial of total abdominal hysterectomy and staging *versus* laparoscopically assisted vaginal hysterectomy and staging for endometrial cancer. Port site metastases in endometrial cancer are less common than in ovarian cancer and, when they occur, are usually in advanced disease.[21]

THE NON-SURGICAL APPROACH

Uncommonly, endometrial cancer may be diagnosed in a nulliparous premenopausal patient who is desirous of preserving fertility. In patients with radiological evidence of stage I disease and with a grade I adenocarcinoma, an alternative treatment strategy is hormonal manipulation. Expert pathological assessment is essential and there must be a thorough hysteroscopic assessment and sampling of endometrial tissue. Wang *et al.*[22] reported on 9 such patients treated with a combination of megestrol acetate, tamoxifen and gonadotrophin-releasing hormone analogue (GnRHa) with 8 patients achieving a complete response. Four patients conceived although in 2 patients this was an ectopic pregnancy, and 5 patients ultimately had a hysterectomy. In our limited experience with these patients, there are often the problems of obesity and reduced possibility of spontaneous or assisted conception.

Montz *et al.*[23] recently reported the use of a progesterone-releasing intra-uterine device in high-risk surgical patients with presumed FIGO stage Ia, grade 1 EEA. The menopausal status of the patients was not given. Patients underwent repeat out-patient endometrial biopsies using the Pipelle. In this small study, the authors reported less morbidity and mortality in these conservatively managed patients compared to a surgically treated matched group. Residual cancer can be detected in these hormonally-treated patients, but pathological responses were also noted. It was not stated for how long conservative treatment should be maintained. The conservative management of EEA cases may, therefore, be appropriate for a highly selected group of patients (stage Ia, grade 1 disease). Repeated anaesthesia is not without risks. In patients with EEA desirous of fertility-preservation, discussion with, and evaluation by, fertility experts is essential.

Also uncommon is the patient who has advanced metastatic disease at presentation, who declines surgery or in whom surgery is considered to be associated with an unacceptable risk. For the patient with advanced disease (*e.g.* with vaginal and lung metastases), it may nevertheless be appropriate to undertake a palliative hysterectomy initially. For the patient who declines surgical treatment or radiation therapy, hormonal treatment can be offered. Care must be exercised in using progestational treatment in patients with cardiac disease. If agreeable, a relatively small dose (*i.e.* palliative dose) of external beam radiotherapy can achieve haemostasis, at least in the short term, when the patient does not wish to undergo a full course of radiotherapy.

A generation ago, it was common to treat endometrial cancer with pre-operative radiotherapy followed by surgery, but this is no longer standard practice. There is also the rare patient who is not a surgical candidate and who is then considered for radiotherapy. However, the results of external beam radiotherapy alone or with brachytherapy similar to that given for cervical cancer yields a less than satisfactory cure rate. Indeed, high-risk surgical patients are also high risk for radiotherapy.

ADJUVANT TREATMENT FOR ENDOMETRIAL ADENOCARCINOMA

This remains a controversial area. On the one hand, it is known that other than grade I stage Ia endometrial cancer, higher grade and higher stage cancers recur and lead to mortality. On the other hand, the value of adjuvant radiotherapy to effect cure or long-term survival in patients remains unproven.[24]

The recently reported PORTEC (Post Operative Radiation Therapy in Endometrial Cancer) study, randomised patients to 46 Gy postoperative external beam radiotherapy (EBRT) or no radiotherapy. Patients had undergone TAH/BSO with no lymph node assessment.[25] There was no difference in survival between the two groups; however, those in the EBRT arm developed fewer locoregional recurrences (4% *versus* 14%). The similarity in survival can be explained by the early detection and treatment of recurrent disease in the group which originally received no radiotherapy. Most recurrences were at the vaginal vault, and could be successfully salvaged. It has been argued that the intensive surveillance in the setting of a trial leads to early pick-up of these recurrences and, therefore, an increased likelihood of successful treatment, which may not be mirrored outside a trial. Importantly, intermediate risk patients only were included (1C grade 1, all grade 2, 1A and 1B grade 3), and so the results cannot be extrapolated to high-risk patients. From multivariate analysis, the authors concluded that postoperative radiotherapy was not indicated in stage 1 patients below 60 years of age and in stage 1B or 1A grade 2 tumours, as the risk of locoregional relapse in this group was 5% or less.

The findings of the randomised Gynecologic Oncology Group (GOG) study #99 included intermediate risk patients who had undergone extensive surgical staging, which were reported in abstract form, concur with the findings of the PORTEC study. Locoregional recurrences were greater in non-irradiated patients, but no significant survival difference was found in the adjuvant-treated group.

For adjuvant radiotherapy, the risks must be balanced against the benefits of reduced local recurrence rates. In a separate paper which looked at the morbidity associated with treatment of endometrial cancer patients in the PORTEC study, Creutzberg et al.[26] found that 26% of the patients in the radiotherapy group suffered late complications compared with 4% in the control group. The severity of the complications were assessed and severe complications, defined as grade 3 (requiring surgery) and grade 4 (leading to death), occurred in 10 patients (3%), all in the radiotherapy group. Patients with acute side-effects were at much greater risk of late complications.

The second arm to the ASTEC trial aims to assess the use of EBRT in high-risk patients irrespective of pelvic node status. High-risk patients are defined as one or more of the following: grade 3 tumours, stage 1C, serous papillary/clear cell type or positive peritoneal cytology. Patients with cervical stromal invasion or positive para-aortic nodes are excluded. Patients may be included in this arm whether or not they have been part of the surgical randomisation.

The role of vaginal brachytherapy (BRT) in endometrial cancer is also unclear. Of interest, this modality of radiotherapy was not used in the GOG #99 or PORTEC studies. A combination of both EBRT and BRT in stage 1 disease may not lead to increased pelvic control or survival, but to a higher rate of complications. Some authors have suggested that brachytherapy alone may have a role in reducing vault recurrences in intermediate risk patients in whom EBRT is not used,[9] with minimal levels of morbidity. However, there have been no randomised trials of this modality. In the PORTEC and GOG #99 studies, the commonest site of recurrence was the vaginal vault. Intuitively, BRT might reduce this risk, whilst causing less morbidity than EBRT. For example, 10.2% of patients in the control arm of the PORTEC study suffered a vaginal relapse, compared with published rates from other studies of patients receiving adjuvant BRT of 2–7%.[25] The authors suggested, therefore, that BRT may reduce the recurrence rate by approximately 50%, but would probably not affect overall survival. For those patient groups in the PORTEC study with a higher 5-year risk of locoregional recurrence without pelvic radiotherapy (aged 60 years or over; stage 1C grades 1 and 2, stage 1B, grade 3), a randomised trial comparing postoperative EBRT alone with BRT alone is planned. This will assess local control, survival, morbidity and quality-of-life.[26] The ASTEC trial allows the use of BRT regardless of the randomisation to EBRT.

In a small number of patients, histology following definitive surgery will reveal stage II disease. In our experience, stage II endometrial cancer is rarely diagnosed before surgery is performed. In cases where there is a pre-operative diagnosis of cervical involvement by endometrial cancer, Mariani et al.[27] reported that a radical hysterectomy alone may be curative in node negative cases. However, there is still debate as to whether the initial treatment should be a radical hysterectomy (alone or with adjuvant radiotherapy) or a simple extrafascial hysterectomy and radiotherapy.[28]

Another clinical dilemma is the patient with disease (EEA) confined to the uterine body but with positive peritoneal cytology. There is one report of an increased incidence of positive peritoneal cytology in patients undergoing laparoscopically assisted vaginal hysterectomy and adenectomy for presumed early stage endometrial cancer.[29] There are also conflicting reports about the clinical importance of positive cytology.[30,31] Management options (in otherwise low stage disease) include an expectant policy, chemotherapy, and follow-up with laparoscopic assessment, which is our favoured approach. Although not popular or in general use in the UK, whole abdominal radiotherapy has also been used.

Hormonal therapy (adjuvant medroxyprogesterone acetate) in high-risk endometrial cancers has been evaluated in the adjuvant setting in a multicentre trial (COSA-NZ-UK) with evidence of a prolonged disease-free interval, but no change in overall survival.[32] However, many patients also had received adjuvant radiotherapy. The authors concluded that adjuvant hormone therapy was not effective in these cancers.

MANAGEMENT OF LESS COMMON ENDOMETRIAL CARCINOMAS

These include CCC, UPSC, adenosquamous cancers, squamous cell cancers and undifferentiated cancers. Although representing only about 10% of endometrial carcinomas, they account for about 50% of relapses in endometrial carcinoma.[33] These rare cancers are characterised by higher stage disease (on surgical/ pathological criteria), more aggressive behaviour (e.g. lymphovascular invasion and lymph node metastases) and worse prognosis. CCC and UPSC should always be considered as poorly differentiated cancers. In part due to their rarity, there is more uncertainty about adjuvant therapy with these cancers than with EEA. The corner-stone of management is surgery but, in almost all cases, adjuvant treatment is recommended as there is usually evidence of high-stage disease. Patients with these cancers should be referred to cancer centres, and surgically managed by gynaecological oncologists. Following surgery for UPSC (and to some extent for CCC), the trend has been to give both pelvic radiotherapy (external beam and vaginal brachytherapy) and platinum-based chemotherapy. Other authors have reported responses to paclitaxel alone or with platinum.[34,35] Other drugs used include doxorubicin, ifosfamide, and cyclophosphamide. UPSC seems to be less chemosensitive than serous papillary ovarian cancer, although commonly considered to be biologically similar to serous papillary cancers of the ovary and peritoneum. In cases of extrapelvic spread of disease, other authors have favoured adjuvant chemo-radiotherapy or whole-abdominal radiotherapy.[36] As all studies have insufficient power and many therapeutic regimens are reported, no evidence-based recommendations can be made as to which are the more efficacious adjuvant treatments.[37] Nevertheless, the survival rates for these cancers remain poor. The interpretation of these studies is undermined by incomplete surgical staging in many surgically treated patients who receive adjuvant treatment.

MANAGEMENT OF ENDOMETRIAL STROMAL SARCOMAS

These rare endometrial cancers are typically described as being either low-grade or high-grade, based on nuclear changes and mitotic rate. ESS represent 10–15% of all uterine sarcomas, which represent about 5% of all uterine cancers. Presentation is usually PMB or irregular perimenopausal bleeding sometimes with pelvic pain. Lymph node sampling or dissection is at the discretion of the surgeon, but the goal of surgery is cytoreduction. Careful histological review is important. Patients require a CT evaluation of chest, abdomen and pelvis. Low-grade ESS (previously referred to as endolymphatic stromal myosis) behaves in an indolent manner but high-grade ESS is usually treated with adjuvant radiotherapy. Interestingly, low grade ESS often express high levels of progesterone receptors which has led to the use of hormonal treatment. Adjuvant treatments rarely impact on overall survival, however.[38] High-grade ESS has a poor prognosis and most cancers will have deep myometrial involvement at initial surgery. As with all gynaecological sarcomas, there is in reality no effective or curative adjuvant treatment for advanced disease although partial and complete responses are reported to some chemotherapy regimens, for example with ifosfamide.[39]

RECURRENT ENDOMETRIAL CANCER

Most recurrences will present within 3 years of initial treatment and most are symptomatic recurrences, challenging the traditional policies of routine vaginal vault smears after surgery and regular follow-up clinics. There is no place for vaginal vault cytology and patients are probably reviewed too frequently after primary treatment. Most recurrences will be in the pelvis, although for the rarer cancers abdominal and chest metastases are frequent even when there has been pelvic control of the disease. With unusual presentations, tissue confirmation of the diagnosis may be important and investigations to document the site(s) of disease are essential. Multidisciplinary team involvement is crucial. The original diagnosis and stage, the treatments and disease-free interval, the extent of the recurrences(s) and the patient's performance status are key factors in the decision making. Ultimately, the treatment emphasis will be either with palliative intent, or less commonly, curative intent.

In patients who have central pelvic disease recurrence after standard surgery and radiotherapy, the only potentially curative procedure is exenterative surgery. Intra-operative radiotherapy may offer some benefit in patients with local recurrence, for example unilateral side wall recurrence who are likely to be left with microscopic disease after surgical excision, although only small case series are available.

ENDOMETRIAL CARCINOMAS

In non-irradiated patients, the usual first line of management of recurrent disease is radiotherapy, although in selected cases further surgery may be undertaken followed by radiotherapy. In many cases with recurrent disease, the patient will have received pelvic radiotherapy. If the radiotherapy was vaginal brachytherapy only, then further radiotherapy can be given as external beam radiotherapy. For central recurrences in the previously irradiated patient in whom no further radiotherapy can be given, exenterative surgery should be considered. A careful metastatic work-up is mandatory. The outlook from exenterative surgery for endometrial carcinoma is, however, less favourable than that for cervical cancer, as extrapelvic disease is more common.

In patients with failed second line treatment or those presenting with widespread metastatic disease, options for treatment include hormonal manipulation with progestational agents, tamoxifen and GnRH agonists, and chemotherapy. Drugs used singly or in combination include platinum, doxorubicin, ifosfamide, cyclophosphamide and paclitaxel. Bony metastases can be treated palliatively by radiotherapy and rarely patients with lung metastases may undergo surgical metastatectomy. Patients presenting with or developing fistulae can undergo palliative diversions and, in general, the simplest surgical procedure should be undertaken. Bowel obstruction is less of a problem with recurrent EC than with ovarian cancer. A gastrostomy tube or PEG tube can provide effective relief of upper abdominal symptoms.[40]

ENDOMETRIAL STROMAL SARCOMA

Low-grade ESS tend to have an indolent course and may present many years later with local pelvic or distant metastases. Surgical extirpation is usually considered the first line of management. It is unclear if surgical extirpation has been successful, whether patients should receive adjuvant treatment – there is little evidence that additional chemotherapy or radiotherapy is of benefit. Hormonal treatment may be of benefit in recurrent disease. High grade ESS often presents with advanced disease, either as disease progression or recurrent disease. Further treatment often involves a combination of modalities with the intent of palliation. Ifosfamide has been reported to have activity in ESS.[39] as has doxorubicin. It should be remembered that an important decision is the decision not to treat, especially in rapidly growing metastatic cancers.

Key points for clinical practice

- Endometrial cancers most often arise from the glandular component and comprise the common endometrioid endometrial adenocarcinoma, and the uncommon, but more lethal, clear cell carcinomas and uterine papillary serous cancers.

Key points for clinical practice (continued)

- Endometrial cancers may also arise from the stroma giving rise to the low-grade and high-grade endometrial stromal sarcomas.

- Generally, endometrial cancers carry a good prognosis, but this is related to early presentation and early stage disease. Stage for stage they are as lethal as other gynaecological cancers and, in particular, less common endometrial cancers have a poor prognosis.

- Management of all but the common endometrioid adenocarcinoma should be undertaken in a cancer centre with assessment by the multidisciplinary team.

- Surgery is the corner-stone of management, but the role and extent of lymph node surgery is unclear. Less common endometrial cancers often have metastatic disease at presentation.

- Laparoscopic and vaginal surgery have a role to play in treatment of endometrioid adenocarcinomas.

- The role of adjuvant radiotherapy is unclear, as is the role of vaginal brachytherapy and external beam pelvic radiotherapy, whole abdominal radiotherapy, chemo-radiotherapy or chemotherapy alone. Rare endometrial cancers are usually more aggressive and adjuvant treatment is recommended despite the lack of evidence of prolonged survival.

- Recurrent disease, if pelvic, can be treated with radiotherapy (if full treatment has not been given previously), exenterative surgery or chemotherapy, but cure is uncommon.

- Extra-abdominal disease is fatal despite combinations of treatment modalities and combination chemotherapy.

- Centralisation of care and large randomised clinical trials may lead to improved non-surgical treatments.

References

1. Anon. *Guidance on Commissioning Cancer Services. Improving Outcomes in Gynaecological Cancers*. London: Department of Health, 1999.
2. Ugwumadu AHN, Carmichael PL, Neven P. Tamoxifen and the female genital tract. *Int J Gynecol Cancer* 1998; **8**: 6–15.
3. Beresford SAA, Weiss NS, Voigt LF, McKnight B. Risk of endometrial cancer in relation to use of oestrogen combined with cyclic progestagen therapy in postmenopausal women. *Lancet* 1997; **349**: 458–461.
4. Women's Health Initiative Randomized Controlled Trial. Risks and benefits of estrogen plus progestin in healthy postmenopausal women. Principal results from the Women's Health Initiative Randomized Controlled Trial. *JAMA* 2002; **288**: 321–333.
5. Anon. *Changing the way we operate. The 2001 Report of the Confidential Enquiry into Perioperative Deaths (NCEPOD)*. London: Department of Health, 2001.
6. Kinkel K, Kaji Y, Yu KK *et al*. Radiologic staging in patients with endometrial cancer: a meta-analysis. *Radiology* 1999; **212**: 711–718.

7. Connor JP, Andrews JI, Anderson B, Buller RE. Computed tomography in endometral carcinoma. *Obstet Gynecol* 2000; **95**: 692–696.
8. Kilgore LC, Partridge EE, Alvarez RD *et al*. Adenocarcinoma of the endometrium: survival comparisons of patients with and without pelvic node sampling. *Gynecol Oncol* 1995; **56**: 29–33.
9. Mohan DS, Samuels MA, Selim MA *et al*. Long-term outcomes of therapeutic pelvic lymphadenectomy for stage I endometrial adenocarcinoma. *Gynecol Oncol* 1998; **70**: 165–171.
10. Naumann RW, Higgins RV, Hall JB. The use of adjuvant radiation therapy by members of the Society of Gynecologic Oncologists. *Gynecol Oncol* 1999; **75**: 4–9.
11. Van Doorn HC, Van Der Zee AGJ, Peeters PHM, Kroeks MVAM, Van Eijkeren MA. Preoperative selection of patients with low stage endometrial cancer at high risk of pelvic lymph node metastases. *Int J Gynecol Cancer* 2002; **12**: 144–148.
12. Orr JWJ, Roland PY, Leichter D, Orr PF. Endometrial cancer: is surgical staging necessary? *Curr Opin Oncol* 2001; **13**: 408–412.
13. Creasman WT, Morrow CP, Bundy BN, Homesley HD, Graham JE, Heller PB. Surgical pathologic spread patterns of endometrial cancer. A Gynecologic Oncology Group Study. *Cancer* 1987; **60**: 2035–2041.
14. Malviya VK, Deppe G, Malone JMJ, Sundareso AS, Lawrence WD. Reliability of frozen section examination in identifying poor prognostic indicators in stage I endometrial adenocarcinoma. *Gynecol Oncol* 1989; **34**: 299–304.
15. Girardi F, Petru E, Heydarfadai M, Haas J, Winter R. Pelvic lymphadenectomy in the surgical treatment of endometrial cancer. *Gynecol Oncol* 1993; **49**: 177–180.
16. Chuang L, Burke, TW, Tornos C *et al*. Staging laparotomy for endometrial carcinoma: assessment of retroperitoneal lymph nodes. *Gynecol Oncol* 1995; **58**: 189–193.
17. Homesley HD, Kadar N, Barrett RJ, Lentz SS. Selective pelvic and periaortic lymphadenectomy does not increase morbidity in surgical staging of endometrial carcinoma. *Am J Obstet Gynecol* 1992; **167**: 1225–1230.
18. Giannice R, Susini T, Ferrandina G *et al*. Systematic pelvic and aortic lymphadenectomy in elderly gynecologic oncologic patients. *Cancer* 2001; **92**: 2562–2566.
19. Morrow CP, Bundy BN, Kurman RJ *et al*. Relationship between surgical-pathological risk factors and outcome in clinical stage I and II carcinoma of the endometrium: a Gynecologic Oncology Group study. *Gynecol Oncol* 1991; **40**: 55–65.
20. Silver DF, Wheeless, Abbas FM. A vaginal extraperitoneal approach to surgically stage patients with endometrial cancer. *Gynecol Oncol* 2001; **81**: 144–149.
21. Manolitsas TP, Fowler JM. Role of laparoscopy in the management of the adnexal mass and the staging of gynecologic cancers. *Clin Obstet Gynecol* 2001; **44**: 495–521.
22. Wang CB, Wang CJ, Huang HJ *et al*. Fertility-preserving treatment in young patients with endometrial adenocarcinoma. *Cancer* 2002; **94**: 2192–2198.
23. Montz FJ, Bristow RE, Bovicelli A, Tomacruz R, Kurman RJ, Intrauterine progesterone treatment of early endometrial cancer. *Am J Obstet Gynecol* 2002; **186**: 651–657.
24. Straughn JM, Huh WK, Kelly FJ *et al*. Conservative management of stage I endometrial carcinoma after surgical staging. *Gynecol Oncol* 2002; **84**: 194–200.
25. Creutzberg CL, van Putten WL, Koper PC *et al*. Surgery and postoperative radiotherapy *versus* surgery alone for patients with stage-1 endometrial carcinoma: multicentre randomised trial. PORTEC Study Group. Post Operative Radiation Therapy in Endometrial Carcinoma. *Lancet* 2002; **355**: 1404–1411.
26. Creutzberg CL, van Putten WL, Koper PC *et al*. The morbidity of treatment for patients with stage I endometrial cancer: results from a randomized trial. *Int J Radiat Oncol Biol Phys* 2001; **51**: 1246–1255.
27. Mariani A, Webb MJ, Keeney GL, Calori G, Podratz KC. Role of wide/radical hysterectomy and pelvic lymph node dissection in endometrial cancer with cervical involvement. *Gynecol Oncol* 2001; **83**: 72–80.
28. Sartori E, Gadducci A, Landoni F *et al*. Clinical behaviour of 203 stage II endometrial cancer cases: the impact of primary surgical approach and of adjuvant radiation therapy. *Int J Gynecol Cancer* 2001; **11**: 430–437.
29. Sonoda Y, Zerbe M, Smith A *et al*. High incidence of positive peritoneal cytology in low-risk endometrial cancer treated by laparoscopically assisted vaginal hysterectomy. *Gynecol Oncol* 2001; **80**: 378–382.

30. Hirai Y, Takeshima N, Kato T, Hasumi K. Malignant potential of positive peritoneal cytology in endometrial cancer. *Obstet Gynecol* 2001; **97**: 725–728.
31. Obermair A, Geramou M, Tripcony L. Peritoneal cytology: impact on disease-free survival in clinical stage I endometrial adenocarcinoma of the uterus. *Cancer Lett* 2001; **164**: 105–110.
32. COSA-NZ-UK Endometrial Cancer Study Groups. Adjuvant medroxyprogesterone acetate in high-risk endometrial cancer. *Int J Gynecol Cancer* 1998; **8**: 387–391.
33. Nguyen NP, Sallah S, Karlsson U *et al*. Prognosis for papillary serous carcinoma of the endometrium after surgical staging. *Int J Gynecol Oncol* 2001; **11**: 305–311.
34. Zanotti KM, Belinson JL, Kennedy AW, Webster KD, Markman M. The use of paclitaxel and platinum-based chemotherapy in uterine papillary serous carcinoma. *Gynecol Oncol* 1999; **74**: 272–277.
35. Ramondetta L, Burk TW, Levenback C *et al*. Treatment of uterine papillary serous carcinoma with paclitaxel. *Gynecol Oncol* 2001; **82**: 156–161.
36. Bancher-Todesca D, Neunteufel W, Williams KE *et al*. Influence of postoperative treatment on survival in patients with uterine papillary serous carcinoma. *Gynecol Oncol* 1998; **71**: 344–335.
37. Tay EH, Ward BG. The treatment of uterine papillary serous carcinoma (UPSC): are we doing the right thing? *Int J Gynecol Cancer* 1999; **9**: 463–469.
38. Bodner K, Bodner-Adler B. Obermair A *et al*. Prognostic parameters in endometrial stromal sarcoma: a clinicopathologic study in 31 patients. *Gynecol Oncol* 2001; **81**: 160–165.
39. Sutton G, Blessing JA, Park R, DiSaia PJ, Rosenshein N. Ifosfamide treatment of recurrent or metastatic endometrial stromal sarcomas previously unexposed to chemotherapy: a study of the Gynecologic Oncology Group. *Obstet Gynecol* 1996; **87**: 747–750.
40. Tsahalina E, Woolas RP, Carter PG *et al*. Gastrostomy tubes in patients with recurrent gynaecological cancer and intestinal obstruction. *Br J Obstet Gynaecol* 1999; **106**: 964–968.

Index